CW00971152

Diabetes, Insulin and the Life of R.D. Lawrence

Jane Lawrence

2012

Diabetes, Insulin and the Life of R.D. Lawrence

Jane Lawrence

Edited by
Robert Tattersall

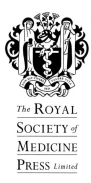

The ROYAL
SOCIETY *of*
MEDICINE
PRESS *Limited*

© 2012 Royal Society of Medicine Press Limited

Published by the Royal Society of Medicine Press Ltd
1 Wimpole Street, London W1G 0AE, UK
Tel: +44 (0)20 7290 2921
Fax: +44 (0)20 7290 2929
E-mail: publishing@rsm.ac.uk
Website: www.rsmpress.co.uk

Apart from any fair dealing for the purposes of research or private study, criticism or review, as permitted under the UK Copyright Designs and Patents Act, 1988, no part of this publication may be reproduced, stored or transmitted, in any form or by any means, without the prior permission in writing of the publishers or in the case of reprographic reproduction in accordance with the terms of licences issued by the Copyright Licensing Agency in the UK, or in accordance with the terms of licences issued by the appropriate Reproduction Rights Organization outside the UK. Enquiries concerning reproduction outside the terms stated here should be sent to the publishers at the UK address printed on this page.

The rights of Jane Lawrence to be identified as author of this work has been asserted by her in accordance with the Copyright, Designs and Patents Act, 1988.

British Library Cataloguing in Publication Data
A catalogue record for this book is available from the British Library

ISBN 978-1-85315-969-5

Distribution in Europe and Rest of World:
Marston Book Services Ltd
PO Box 269
Abingdon
Oxon OX14 4YN, UK
Tel:+44 (0)1235 465500
Fax: +44 (0)1235 465555
Email: direct.order@marston.com

Distribution in the USA and Canada:
Royal Society of Medicine Press Ltd
c/o BookMasters, Inc
30 Amberwood Parkway
Ashland, Ohio 44805, USA
Tel: +1 800 247 6553 / +1 800 266 5564
Email: order@bookmasters.com

Typeset by Phoenix Photosetting, Chatham, Kent, UK
Printed and bound by Replika Press Pvt. Ltd, India

Contents

Dedication

To the memory of Anna Lawrence, without whom RDL would not have had such a happy life or such a successful career.

AGL

Contributors

Judith Allsop BSc (Econ), MSc (Econ), PhD, Cert.Ed.
Visiting Professor of Health Policy,
University of Lincoln,
Lincoln

Harry Keen CBE MD FRCP
Hon. President, International Diabetes Federation,
Hon. Vice President Diabetes UK
Emeritus Professor of Human Metabolism and Consultant Physician
Guy's Hospital Campus, King's College, London
Warwick University Medical School, Warwick

Jane Lawrence B.Ed (Hons)
Retired Headteacher,
Sheen Mount Primary School,
London

Robert Tattersall BA MA MD FRCP
Retired Professor of Clinical Diabetes,
University of Nottingham,
Nottingham

Peter J Watkins, MD, FRCP
Consultant Physician (retired),
Kings College Hospital,
London

Alex D Wright MA, MB BChir, FRCP, FRCP(C)
Consultant Diabetologist,
Selly Oak Hospital;
Senior Lecturer in Medicine and Foundation Fellow,
University of Birmingham,
Birmingham

Foreword

I first met Robin Lawrence by chance when in 1952 I went to a symposium in London organised by the CIBA pharmaceutical company. At the time there was no treatment for diabetic retinopathy and some young diabetics were going blind. One of the talks was by two Swedish doctors, Rolf Luft a physician and Herbert Olivekrona a neurosurgeon who had undertaken the surgical removal of the pituitary gland, a fairly perilous procedure, as a form of treatment for sight-threatening retinopathy. They showed a series of before and after retinal photographs which purported to show improvement. In the silence that followed their talk, I heard a loud hurrumphing a couple of rows behind me and turned to see a distinguished looking, silver haired man with a high collar and a carnation in his button hole stating in a very loud sotto voce 'I'd want my eyes to look a lot better than that if I was having my pituitary out!' 'That's R D Lawrence' said my colleague.

My research task at the time was to explore a recently published suggestion that not only did people with diabetes have high blood pressure but so too did their close but non-diabetic relatives. My chief, George Pickering (later Sir George), was a blood pressure expert and set me the task of measuring the blood pressure of all the diabetic patients at St Mary's Hospital and their first degree relatives. After a few weeks I found that though we had lots of older, diet-treated patients (there were no tablets then) at St Mary's, we were very short of younger, insulin-dependent patients. 'That's because they all go to Kings to see Lawrence' explained Pickering, 'He's the best thing King's ever had!' and sent me off to see him with a little explanatory note.

So began my relationship with RDL, which started quite properly as master and boy and matured through professional collegiacy into warm, personal friendship. I ushered him away for coffee and biscuits when he got hypoglycaemic seeing patients in the Clinic, was introduced by him to Elliot P Joslin and Charles Best and was a guest at what I think must have been his 70th birthday dinner. I distinguished myself by loudly declaring that I thought the troubled NHS (when was it not?) should be run by that very efficient Sainsbury's and the guest beside me said 'Do you really believe that?' 'Yes' I said with more force than I felt. 'And you didn't know I was Lady Sainsbury?' she asked. Despite his great celebrity he was a refreshingly non-conformist, even radical character. He distinguished himself – in my eyes at least – as being, with Alec Bourne – the only outspoken supporters of a National Health Service when this was almost a heresy in Harley Street.

What also impressed me as a young doctor was the understanding and sympathy he showed for his young patients and this shines through in the practicality and humanity of *The Diabetic Life*, his book for patients **and** doctors. He taught newly diagnosed patients about diet himself. He would not have dietitians in the Clinic. 'If the doctor can't teach it, the patients won't understand it' he averred. Every diabetic his own doctor – one of his adages – set my course on patient empowerment for a lifetime.

My last clear recollection was, after his stroke, when I drove him to the annual diabetic childrens Christmas party at King's College Hospital when he insisted on using his walking support as a hockey stick and batting an orange around the hall to the delight of the children. That scene is a fitting end to a Foreword to the story of a great life which follows and which contributed to many new hope and some delivery from the tyranny of diabetes.

Harry Keen CBE MD FRCP

Preface

All doctors who attend meetings of the medical and scientific section of Diabetes UK know the name of Dr RD (Robin) Lawrence, through the RD Lawrence fellowship which supports young researchers and the RD Lawrence lecture which has been awarded since 1973 to clinical or non clinical researchers under age 45. What they may not know is that Lawrence founded the Diabetic Association, precursor of Diabetes UK, in 1934 and was a prime mover in establishing the International Diabetes Federation of which he became the first chairman in 1950. His name is also perpetuated at King's College Hospital were he spent his working life. King's has an RD Lawrence ward and more recently has endowed an RD Lawrence chair of diabetic medicine.

From these tributes, the young diabetologist will conclude that he was a great man but what exactly did he do to deserve such recognition?

After his election as President of the Students' Representative Council at Aberdeen University in 1914, the student paper commented on 'his personal qualities of, 'a frank and open manner, which, combined with a belief in himself, makes others put their confidence in him. Self-reliant, independent to a degree, he is none the less one of the most companionable fellows one could ever wish to meet… Fortunately, he is blessed with a sense of humour which allows him to laugh at himself: and his dignity is not a thing which bothers him much, when it is convenient to forget about it.' This article also mentioned his sporting and musical talents and concluded that he would go far.

Professionally, Lawrence did in England what Elliott Joslin did in the USA – shaped the clinical management of diabetes for nearly 40 years. Like Joslin, he put patients centre stage and insisted that they were in charge of looking after their disease. Unlike most physicians who treated diabetes at London teaching hospitals he was a hands on doctor who talked to patients in language they could understand and set them achievable targets. Having diabetes himself meant that he indulged in personal crusade to improve the lives of diabetics with whom he felt a deep kinship. In 1925, he produced the first edition of the enduringly popular and practical, *The Diabetic Life: Its control by diet and insulin*, which reached its 17th edition in 1965 and was translated into many languages.

This biography presents a comprehensive picture of the extraordinarily full life of a great man.

Robert Tattersall
March 2012

Acknowledgements

At a Lawrence's centenary dinner in December 1992 I met J. G. L. Jackson known as Jim, (1923–2002) who was working on Lawrence's biography. Jim had worked with Lawrence and contributed to the founding of European Association for the Study of Diabetes (EASD) and IDF. He was Secretary-General of BDA (1954), the first Executive Director of EASD (1970–1988) and Secretary-in-Chief of IDF (1957–1960). For many early years he was described as 'the heart, soul and engine house' of the BDA and also played a key role in the foundation and establishment of the IDF.

Before his death in 2002, Jim had published four accounts of Lawrence's work in *Diabetic Medicine* which were later published by the *Wiley Online Library*. These included R. D. Lawrence, H. G. Wells, G. B. Shaw: A Vignette, R. D. Lawrence and the Formation of the Diabetic Association, The formation of the medical and scientific section of the British Diabetic Association and R. D. Lawrence: a father of international diabetes. Jackson had drawn together biographical material from *A Splendid Life* which was Lawrence's draft notes for his autobiography. I am deeply indebted to all the work he did on my father-in-law's life and work.

I had just completed writing up my own family history in 2006 and was keen to begin another project. Adam Lawrence agreed to let me write his father's biography and I would like to thank all those who have helped me. Dr Mike Williams in Aberdeen had campaigned successfully for the erection of a plaque at Lawrence's nearby birthplace. He was enormously helpful to me and showed me round Aberdeen taking me to all the places familiar to Lawrence. We spent many hours in the University's Special Libraries and Archives researching Lawrence's university years and he read through and corrected early drafts of the opening chapters.

Nancy Jackson and Harry Keen were particularly supportive and helpful. Dr Peter Watkins provided a sheaf of material from KCH and also much encouragement and also he enabled us to meet at the RSM for discussions about the project. By a fortuitous quirk of fate I was put in touch Dr Alex Wright who had developed a lifelong interest in Lawrence having worked with him at KCH. He has been a huge source of support throughout and drew together a team to work on the medical and scientific side of Lawrence's career. He introduced me to Professor Robert Tattersall who has been a very supportive editor working with unfailing professionalism and patience with me as the chapters flew back and forth between us.

Thanks to my friend and fellow walker Judy de Gory who in her professional capacity as Professor Judith Allsop was very encouraging when energy for the project flagged and she wrote the chapter on *Speaking Out – the Formation of the*

Diabetic Association. The late Professor Keith Taylor who had worked with Lawrence added many personal insights and offered welcome support and encouragement.

Many thanks to the Scottish Society for History of Medicine (the Guthrie Trust), the Diabetes Research Fund and to Novo Nordisk for providing financial support for the project for the project and also to Diabetes UK who allowed me to roam freely in their archive as well as providing financial support and answering a string of queries.

Thanks to Dan and Adam Lawrence for their generosity with funds for the project and to my family for their encouragement and support. Particular thanks to my brother-in-law John Morrell for his patience and accuracy when proof reading the early drafts.

Jane Lawrence
March 2012

CHAPTER 1

A Stroke of Luck

In January 1920, a Scottish doctor, Robert Daniel Lawrence, was appointed second House Surgeon in the Casualty Department of King's College Hospital. It was unusual for a London teaching hospital to appoint outsiders, but Lawrence, known to his friends as Robin, had a shelf of gold medals from his student days in Aberdeen and had passed the primary part of the Fellowship of the Royal College of Surgeons (FRCS) as a second-year medical student. His ambition was to become a professor of surgery. He must have impressed the powers at King's, because, after his 6-month stint in casualty, he was told he could apply for any job as if he were a King's man. He became assistant surgeon in the Ear, Nose and Throat (ENT) Department. In November 1920, while practising a mastoidectomy on a corpse in the mortuary, a chip of bone flew into his eye, which became, in his words, 'violently septic'. In a talk in 1961, Lawrence said, 'It was my habit to go to the PM room at night and dissect the trouble that had gone wrong and find out why they had died, and then practise the operation on the other side. Some might think this gruesome. I had no time for thoughts of that sort.' However, Theodore Whittington, then an ophthalmology house surgeon at King's, thought that to take himself off to the post-mortem room was 'quite wrong, but typical of Lawrence in his experimental fashion, and probably nothing had been sterilized and he was probably not particularly expert.' Whittington remembered how his boss Vernon Cargill (1866–1955), an eminent and influential opthalmologist who had been Lord Lister's house surgeon,[A] came down to Out Patients and told Whittington how worried he was about a corneal wound in an eye of one of the residents.[B] In those pre-antibiotic days, the only treatment for sepsis in the eye was to wash it out. This was a painful business, but worse followed when the sister on night duty tested his urine and found it was loaded with sugar. The next day, the biochemist, Dr Geoffrey Arthur Harrison, did a blood sugar and found it to be three times normal.[C]

The prognosis of diabetes at this time depended on the age of the patient. In his 1866 book, *Diabetes: Its Various Forms and Different Treatments*, the English physician George Harley (1829–1896) suggested that there were two types.[1] In one,

A. Whittington recalled Cargill saying, 'When I die, I want it written on my tombstone, nothing else, HE WAS LORD LISTER'S HOUSE SURGEON.'
B. Personal letter from Whittington to RDL, 17 November 1962.
C. The sugar in the blood is glucose and today doctors always talk about blood glucose. However, during Lawrence's lifetime, they all talked of blood sugar.

the sufferer was 'fat and ruddy', which Harley attributed to excessive formation of sugar by the liver. The other was due to an inability to use food, with emaciation one of the earliest and most prominent symptoms. These corresponded to what in the 1880s a French physician Etienne Lancereaux (1829–1910) called *diabète gras* (fat) and *diabète maigre* (thin) – which now we call types 2 and 1. The first clue that they might have different causes came in 1889 when Oskar Minkowski (1858–1931) discovered serendipitously that removing the pancreas of a dog caused a severe wasting type of diabetes.[2] Most physiologists thought this was because the pancreas, or more specifically a group of specialized cells, the islands of Langerhans, produced an internal secretion that controlled carbohydrate metabolism. By 1920, this hypothetical internal secretion or hormone even had a name. In 1909, a Belgian physiologist Jean de Meyer (1878–1934) called it insuline. Unfortunately, attempts between 1890 and 1920 to cure severe diabetes by feeding or injecting animal pancreatic extracts had been an abject failure. Possible explanations were that there was no internal secretion or, if there was, it was not stored in the pancreas or that beef or other animal insulins did not work in humans.

Lawrence's parents were not medical, but they would surely have looked up diabetes in a reference book such as the *Harmsworth Universal Encyclopaedia*, where they would have been dismayed to read that:

As the disease progresses, the patient generally loses weight, the skin becomes dry, and the tongue red and glazed. Under treatment the condition may be much improved and life prolonged for many years, though complete and permanent cure is rare. Death may result from gradual exhaustion, or from the accumulation of a poison in the blood which gives rise to a condition of profound unconsciousness known as diabetic coma, or the patient may develop tuberculosis or die from pneumonia. Complications which may arise are inflammation of the kidneys, neuritis, paralysis, affections of the eye, and changes in the skin. The essential factor in the treatment is regulation of the diet so as to reduce to an absolute minimum sugar and starchy foods. Drug treatment is of little avail. A recent form of treatment in which the patient fasts more or less completely has given encouraging results.

The recent form of treatment referred to was the notorious starvation diet of the American physician Frederick Madison Allen (1876–1964), which had been described in great detail in 1919 in a book, *Total Dietary Regulation in the Treatment of Diabetes*.[3] The rationale of Allen's treatment was animal experiments in which he removed varying amounts of the pancreas to produce the equivalents of mild or severe human diabetes. Dogs with 20% of their pancreas or more left did not develop diabetes. The fate of those with 80–90% of their pancreas removed depended on what they ate. A daily average intake adult of carbohydrate is between 150 and 300 g per day. On a low-carbohydrate diet, they remained relatively well, like middle-aged humans with diabetes. Allen called this an Eskimo diet, since Eskimos lived on only 52 g of carbohydrate daily. Large amounts of carbohydrate (a Hindu diet) wore out the pancreas and what had originally been mild diabetes turned into the severe pancreatic form. However, if the same animals were fed a high-fat diet, the amount of glucose in the urine (glycosuria) disappeared or was greatly reduced. From this, Allen decreed that diabetics should order their lives 'according to the size of their pancreas', which basically meant reducing the amount of food until glycosuria disappeared. The first fact that Allen demonstrated to his own satisfaction was that, on fasting, even the most severe cases of human diabetes became free from glycosuria and were often less acidotic as well. The basis of his method was complete starvation for 10 days on a diet of:

Water	*1500–2000 cc [cm³] per day*
Coffee	*1–3 cups*
Clear meat soup up to 600 cc	
Bran muffins [to produce satiety and combat constipation] 3–6	

After the urine had become sugar-free, the next stage was to determine the patient's carbohydrate tolerance. Vegetables were added and the amount gradually increased until sugar reappeared in the urine. At this point, carbohydrate was decreased and protein added up to 1.5 g per kg. Finally, fat was added until the calorific value of the diet was 'sufficient'. Dietary restriction had been the basis of diabetes treatment for more than a century, but the novel aspect of Allen's treatment was his insistence that the severest diabetics should be kept permanently underweight. The previous philosophy had been that, after glycosuria had been abolished by fasting, the patient should be fattened up by adding as many non-carbohydrate calories as possible, weight gain being the sign of success

The most enthusiastic advocate of Allen's treatment was Elliott Proctor Joslin (1869–1962) of Boston, who became the most famous diabetes specialist of the twentieth century and whose textbook went through 10 editions in his lifetime. Lawrence wrote:

When I began to read about diabetes and the Allen treatment and the great book of Joslin (because Joslin was the English book which everybody read in those days), and when he said, in the 1919 edition, that by the Allen treatment of starving on a very low diet you might live three years with luck, and in the 1920 edition he said four years with luck, I found that was very depressing.

To stick to Allen's diet as an outpatient needed enormous courage and determination. Many physicians thought the treatment was cruel and some patients stated frankly that death was preferable to the agonies of starvation. In 1921, John R. Williams (1874–1965), Chief of Medicine at the Highlands Hospital, Rochester, New York, claimed that most failures were due to 'unfaithfulness on the part of the patient', and a chart in his paper purports to show that of 73 deaths in patients with severe diabetes, 46 came about because the treatment had been abandoned. He commented that 'many cases unquestionably die because of lack of courage'.[4] For many 'faithful' patients, the result of the regimen was literal starvation, and some patients died of inanition not diabetes. In 1921, the famous German diabetes specialist Carl von Noorden (1858–1944) turned away in disapproval when he saw Joslin's prize patient, 17-year-old Ruth A, who at just over five feet weighed only 54 lb (24.5 kg): a body mass index (BMI) of less than 14 kg/m^2. Irrespective of whether they 'cheated', the survival of patients on the Allen diet must also have depended on intrinsic factors such as the rate of destruction of the insulin-producing cells and extrinsic factors such as infections.

There was an expert on dietary treatment of diabetes in London, George Graham (1882–1971) at Barts, but there is no evidence that Lawrence consulted him. Probably he did not need to, since the biochemist at King's who had diagnosed his diabetes, Geoffrey Harrison (1894–1982), was already doing research on diabetes. In March 1921, in a grant application to the Medical Research Council (MRC), Harrison wrote of his method:

> Each patient is made 'sugar free' (if possible) by starvation. The 'working tolerance' is then determined separately for carbohydrates, proteins and fats, using common everyday foods, the aim being to render each patient 'sugar free' and 'acetone body' [free] … with the maximum calorific value per kilogram.

The most Lawrence could hope for was a much shortened life on a rigid diet, and, realizing that a career in surgery was now impossible, he turned instead to laboratory medicine. This must have been a bitter blow, as his heart had been set on surgery for many years. In January 1921, he took up a post in the biochemistry laboratory at King's and began work on an MD thesis with the support of Harrison. This was an era when an equable climate was thought to aid recuperation from virtually any disease, and this is probably why Lawrence was given three months' leave of absence, which he spent first in the subtropical town of Menton on the French Riviera and then in Italy. Letters to his parents described warm sun, clear blue skies and many outings in delightful company, but nothing about diabetes or any inconveniences imposed by his new regime. He did, however, mention that he was still nearly blind in his left eye.

He returned to King's for the summer of 1921 and was seen in a punt raising awareness of an extreme bed shortage at the hospital. Throughout the autumn of 1921, he worked on his thesis *The Estimation of Diastase in Blood and Urine and its Diagnostic Significance*.[5]

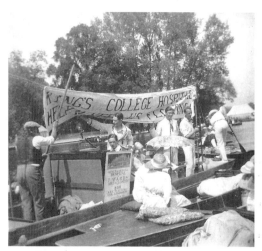

His health must have remained reasonably good, as he took a skiing holiday in Villars over Christmas and New Year of 1921–22. Photographs show him to be fit, active and doing cross-country skiing on un-pisted slopes, a notoriously tough activity, especially on a severely restricted diet. He continued work on the thesis in the spring of 1922 and was awarded his MD in March, returning to Aberdeen for the graduation ceremony.

King's College Hospital, 1921. 'Help to Keep us Floating'.

Lawrence did not know about it

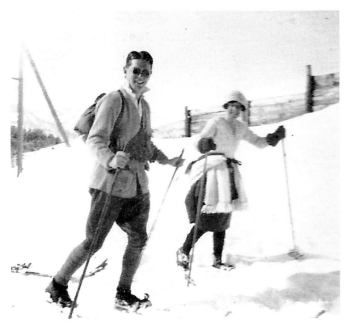

There were no lifts or beautifully groomed pistes in Villars in 1921.

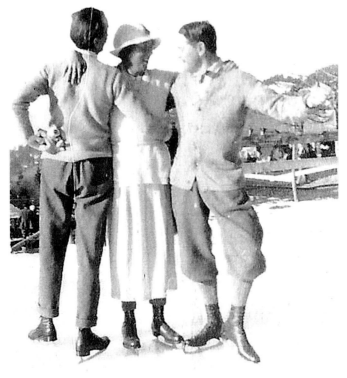

The Three Graces, Spring 1921. Lawrence RH.

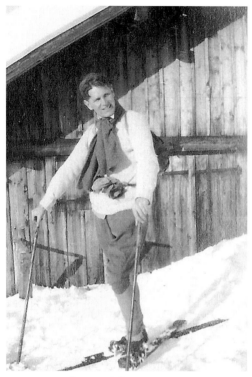

Lawrence: Looking good for one living on the Allen diet.

yet, but in early 1922 a momentous discovery had been made in far-off Canada. The definitive account of how insulin was discovered in Toronto by Frederick Banting (1891–1941) and Charles Best (1899–1978) in the department of the Aberdeen-born professor of physiology J. J. R. Macleod (1876–1935) has been written by Michael Bliss.[6] The first use of insulin (a pancreatic extract made by Best) on a human was on 11 January 1922 when the house physician at Toronto General Hospital, Ed Jeffery, injected 15 cc of what he described as 'thick brown muck' into the buttocks of 14-year-old Leonard Thompson, who had been on the Allen diet since 1919 and weighed only 65 lb (29.5 kg). Banting did not have treatment rights at the hospital and therefore the test was directed by Dr Walter Campbell (1891–1981), who chose Thompson because, 'We thought it should be tried on the most severe cases we could find, for two reasons. If nothing happened their number was up anyway, and, more important, if effective in such patients, the results could not be gainsaid.'[7]

After the injection, Thompson's blood sugar fell from 24.4 to 18.3 mmol/L, but there was no clinical benefit and he developed a sterile abscess at one of the injection sites. This test was obviously a failure, but treatment resumed on 23 January, when he was given 5 cc of a new extract prepared by the biochemist J. B. (Bert) Collip (1892–1965) and then 10 cc more over the next 24 hours. This time, the results were spectacular. Thompson's blood sugar fell from 29 mmol/L on the morning of 29 January to 6.7 mmol/L at 5 am the next morning. He continued on

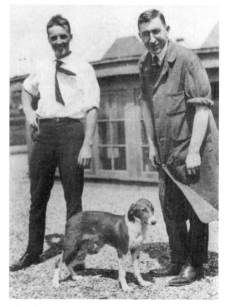

The discovery of insulin by Frederick Banting and Charles Best.

Collip's potent extract for the next 10 days, with marked clinical improvement and complete elimination of his glycosuria and ketonuria. The first clinical results were published in the March 1922 issue of the *Canadian Medical Association Journal* where the authors reported that, up to 22 February, they had treated seven cases, Leonard Thompson being the only one described in detail. Dramatically, the paper drew the following conclusions:[8]

(i)   Blood sugar could be markedly reduced, even to normal values.
(ii)   Glycosuria could be abolished.
(iii) The acetone bodies could be made to disappear from the urine.
(iv)   The respiratory quotient showed evidence of increased utilization of carbohydrates.
(v)   A definite improvement was observed in the general condition of these patients and, in addition, the patients themselves reported a subjective sense of wellbeing and increased vigour for a period following the administration of these preparations.

In Toronto, production was handed over to the Connaught Laboratories, a small industrial plant set up in 1914 to make vaccines and antitoxins, but its first efforts between February and May 1922 were dogged by problems. It was therefore decided to call in Eli Lilly and Co. of Indianapolis, a company with experience in production and standardization of glandular extracts. The Dean of the University

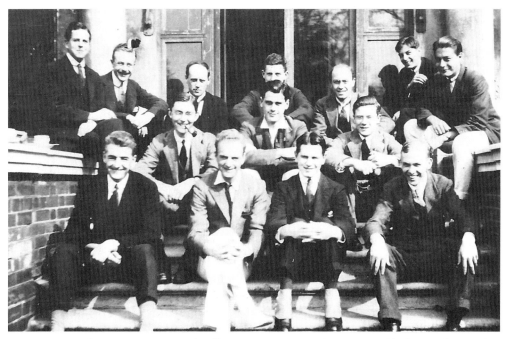

Lawrence, centre front wearing spats, with colleagues at KCH September 1921 outside the large house called Platances on Denmark Hill where they lodged.

of Toronto set up an 'insulin committee' to manage the problems of the patent, finances and monitoring the quality of insulin. At the end of May, the University gave Lilly exclusive rights to produce and sell insulin for one year. Lilly's part of the bargain was to provide free insulin for clinical trials to selected clinicians in North America (whom Lilly's research director later described as 'the insulin aristocrats'), to have all batches tested in Toronto and to assign the patent for any improvements to the University.

It is not clear when Lawrence and Harrison heard about the discovery of insulin, but the first announcement in the medical literature in Britain was on 22 July 1922, when the *British Medical Journal* (*BMJ*) printed an annotation that reviewed the theoretical basis of the discovery and the effect of the extract on blood sugar in dogs.[9] The writer hoped that 'before long sufficient clinical results will be forthcoming to show whether the sanguine expectations the Toronto observations will raise are well founded'. Presumably, it was in response to this that Harrison wrote on 24 July to Lawrence's old University friend A. Landsborough Thompson, secretary of the Medical Research Council (MRC), saying, 'I should like to see you sometime re question of possible supply of pancreatic islet tissue for treatment tests on some of my diabetics under dietetic control.'

Landsborough Thomson replied asking whether Harrison wanted to make his own pancreatic extract or whether he hoped to get supplies of insulin from Toronto. In the event, Harrison was disappointed, because he was not chosen to participate in the subsequent MRC trial of insulin. In July 1922, the University of Toronto asked if the MRC would accept the patent rights of a pancreatic extract known as insulin.[10] The Council was doubtful, but eventually agreed to take it on. The renowned physiologist Henry Dale (1875–1968) and his biochemist colleague Harold Dudley (1889–1935) went to North America to find out the facts. At Eli Lilly in Indianapolis, they were shown the still rather crude large-scale production process. In their report to the MRC, they concluded:[11]

> *In general, the manufacture of the extract, both in Toronto and Indianapolis, is in a very unsatisfactory state. The yield is below that obtained in small scale experiments and is very irregular, sometimes a potent and sometimes a very weak end product results, and the reasons for these frequent failures are not known. ... Just before we left America, both the Eli Lilly Co. and the Toronto laboratory were in great difficulty owing to the fact that their products were proving to be unstable, the potency falling off to practically nothing in a week.*

Dale was worried that the Toronto patent seemed too vague and general. However, the great clamour for insulin from physicians and the public meant that the MRC had to do something, and one advantage would be that they could 'exercise a moral control of manufacturers and induce them to submit to a system of supervision, as regards this product, which the law does not enable the Council at present to enforce'. The reason the MRC had no power was that, until the passing of the Therapeutic Substances Act in 1925, any drug could be advertised and marketed as a cure for any disease even if it was completely ineffective.

It was probably in the summer of 1922 that Lawrence's health deteriorated.

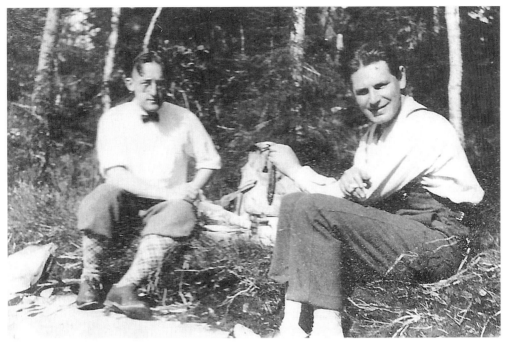

Outings in Tuscany with Dino Spranger.

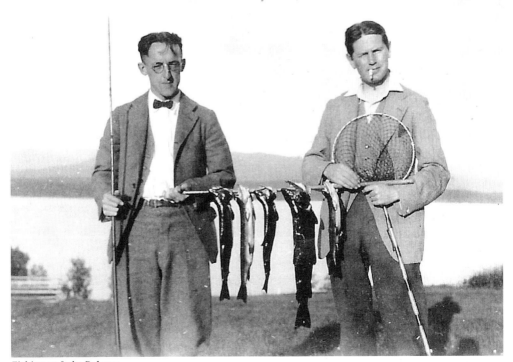

Fishing at Lake Bolsena.

He noticed that whenever he worked particularly hard, his diabetes got worse. Realizing the hopeless prognosis, he gave up any notion of working hard at King's. The easiest course of action would have been to go home to Aberdeen to be cared for by his mother, but he said that 'one thing I wouldn't do was to go home and die, with all the anxiety and horrid tension in one's own home'. The tension and distress would arise with all the waiting while he was in his terminal phase of starvation and coma. Lawrence found a bold solution to what he must have thought would be the last major decision of his life. He was thin, his eyes were very sensitive to light and he felt the cold. He later wrote:

I set about trying to get an easy life for myself. I was advised by the chief, Sir St Clair Thompson [1853–1943], a very famous throat man in the ENT department, that I should go to Florence and be a general practitioner there. In his earlier life as a doctor he had tubercle, and went there to practise. He got better, and then became this famous man at King's and all over the country. He gave me lots of introductions to people he had still kept up with, saying that there were six English speaking doctors before the First World War and none afterwards. So there was an opening for me he said. So off I set to Florence with a dictionary, a stethoscope, and Gulliver's Travels in Italian. That is the best way to learn a language – get a book you know fairly well in English, translated. I wanted to take the Bible, but it wasn't well translated into Italian, and so I thought Gulliver's Travels was very much better. I got on fairly well there and I was quite fortunate. I got a good consulting room in the main street, and began to get patients. I was pretty fit, good tolerance [for food], and I was able to play tennis and dance, and things like that, and life wasn't too bad. I think I earned enough money not to use up all my capital. I had a wonderful capital from the First World War – a gratuity of about £500.

Things went well at first:

I was pretty fit and well, and enjoying life and the art of Florence, until I got bronchitis. And then downhill as always happens; got full of sugar and acetone; lost weight; got so weak that I couldn't walk upstairs and I would fall down, and altogether things were getting pretty horrid. I would even fall asleep when interviewing a new patient. That tells you how bad I was with the acetone. A new patient in those days to me was a terrific event, and they were not plentiful. There were a lot of English residents there, and travelling English ate most unsuitable food and drank far too much Chianti, and so they needed my attention very frequently.

We do not know whether Lawrence received the *BMJ* in Italy, but Harrison certainly read it in London. On 4 November 1922, it contained an article by Banting's boss J. J. R. Macleod in which he wrote that sufficient human cases had been treated to 'justify the statement that when insulin is administered subcutaneously in adequate dosage it is capable, within a remarkably short time, of removing the cardinal symptoms of the disease for a period of several hours. To suppress the symptoms permanently, however, the injections must be repeated, the practice at present being twice daily. So long as the administration is maintained the patient is able to assimilate much more carbohydrate than previously, and he gains weight and with it both physical and mental vigour.'[12]

Two weeks later the *BMJ* published a statement by the MRC emphasizing that insulin was not yet available in Britain but that they were organizing 'a thorough and scientific trial of the new treatment in this country'. Insulin would be tested at seven teaching hospitals, where investigators undertook to work 'as members of a coordinated team in close touch with the National Institute for Medical Research, with a view to achieving the most rapid progress possible towards improved methods of preparing and using the extract'.[13] One unforeseen consequence of the MRC's involvement was that for the first time they were exposed to the pathos of severe illness and 'inquiring, appealing, often heartrending letters arrived by the sackful, so that ordinary correspondence became submerged'. The MRC refused to give insulin to anyone who was not participating in their trials. Thus, for example, William Ralph Inge (1860–1954), the Dean of St Paul's, nicknamed the gloomy dean for his general pessimism, was denied treatment for his 13-year-old daughter Paula, who died.

On 6 January 1923 the *BMJ* published an article on further clinical experience with insulin by Banting and two Toronto clinicians, Walter Campbell and Andrew Almon Fletcher.[14] They reported that:

Up to the present time fifty cases have been treated with insulin, and some have been under treatment continuously for several months. Although the most striking results have been seen in children and young adults, all patients have been benefited by the treatment. Many of the patients have come to the hospital in a state of extreme under-nutrition, suffering from great weakness along with an indisposition to any physical activity. On the first or second day of treatment, if sufficient insulin

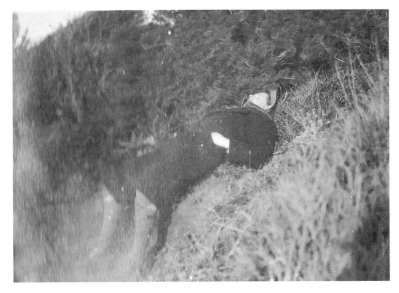

Lawrence, Spring 1923, sleepy and feeling the cold.

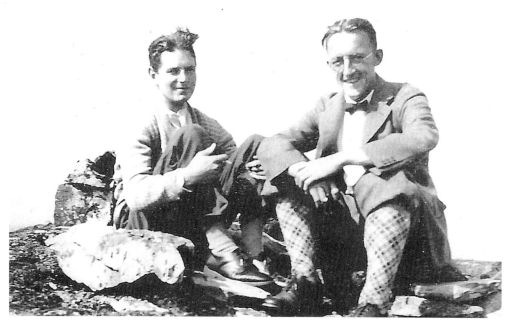

Lawrence holding a cigarette with difficulty because of his peripheral neuritis.

is given, the urine becomes sugar-free, and on the second or third day ketone-free. These patients become conscious of increasing strength before the end of the first week.

Readers of the *BMJ* were doubtless amazed to learn that some patients had been well enough after a month to go back to work. Meanwhile in Florence, Lawrence cut his diet, especially carbohydrates, to the barest minimum:

Breakfast, no bread or rolls; cheese, lettuce, celery, olives, black coffee. The meat and vegetable meals at lunch and dinner were tolerable, especially when a glass of dry Chianti wine was added; this gave a little energy, as the French physicians of the eighteenth century had found when they prescribed a litre per day of vin ordinaire.

But despite this rigid regime, his urine was still full of sugar and a dangerous amount of ketones, the breakdown product of fat. Luckily, there was a lift in his lodgings, so he struggled on, but by now he was receiving only the merest trickle of new patients. It was probably after reading the January article that Geoffrey Harrison wrote about the results of insulin treatment in Canada and suggested that Lawrence should go there. Lawrence remembered later that his reaction was:

I had had so many disappointments by trying quack remedies that I wrote back without enthusiasm saying I would wait and see, without feeling any optimism. But when peripheral neuritis was added to the other troubles, so that I could not handle a match to light the solacing cigarette, I felt that the struggle to keep alive – it could not be called living – was no longer tolerable nor worth while, although Florence had some beautiful sedentary compensations in architecture, pictures and music.

His scepticism was shared by many others. An editorialist in the *Lancet* in August 1922 seems to have been under the impression that the extract had to be given intravenously two or three times a day so that 'the widespread application of the treatment in its present form is not very practicable'. It is said that in 1922 the premier German diabetes specialist Bernard Naunyn wrote to his former pupil Oskar Minkowski telling him not to believe a word of it as it was another case of American bluff.

On 24 February 1923, an annotation in the *BMJ* reported that the MRC had made 'rapid and satisfactory progress' in its trial, although insulin was not yet generally available.[15] No date was given for when it would be. Eventually, on 21 April 1923, the BMJ contained a statement from the MRC headed 'INSULIN AVAILABLE IN THIS COUNTRY' [capitals in the original].[16] The suppliers were British Drug Houses and Burroughs Wellcome, and it was expected that insulin from three other British firms would soon become available, as well as a consignment from Eli Lilly in Indianapolis. Insulin was only to be released to hospitals that had blood-sugar measuring facilities and was only to be given to diabetics whose symptoms could not be controlled with moderate dietary restriction. In the words of the communiqué, there was to be 'no luxury use of insulin until supplies are abundant'. In fact, the cost would have discouraged luxury use. Insulin came in rubber-capped bottles of 100 or 200 units costing 25 and 50 shillings, respectively. To put these prices in context, the wages of the average worker were £180 a year and a dozen large bottles of port cost 50s 0d.

Hospitals and practitioners wanting an immediate supply were enjoined to apply to one of the two British firms, and this is presumably what Harrison did before sending a telegram to Lawrence telling him, 'I've got some insulin come back quick it works.'

On 10 May 1923, when Lawrence probably only had a few weeks left to live, he wrote to Harrison:

I am going to try to get home and have a fortnight with you before you go on holiday. I hope you can find me a bed somewhere there: perhaps you have now got a bit of a ward for your diabetics. I don't seem able to free myself of sugar (+++) on a small diet and have got distinct numbness of fingers and feet – peripheral neuritis – so I think it is time to give in here and run away from what patients I have left. If I don't hear from you to the contrary, I shall turn up letting you know the exact date as soon as I can. I want to bring my motor home; sounds opulent doesn't it, but my banker hardly would think so. So you'll see me as soon as I can get there. I'm a damned

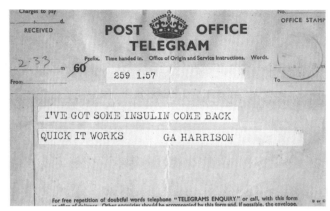

Telegram from Dr Harrison (not the original).

nuisance to myself and my friends, I know, but que voulez-vous? *I shall be greatly interested in your insulin work and look forward to talks.*

Six days later, he wrote a cheery and stoical letter to Harrison again just before his departure:

I am leaving here soon and shall turn up on Monday, 28th May, starving before breakfast. I am looking forward to the treatment very much and have assumed that I shall be benefited, so shall be very bad-tempered if it doesn't work. I don't like peripheral neuritis. It interferes with work. Cheerio. Till then, Yours RDL.

Lawrence described his epic drive of nearly 1000 miles across Italy and France as 'a pretty tough journey'. This was an understatement. His chauffeur was an Italian garage man who wanted to go to England to see his son, who ran a restaurant in Soho. They drove in Lawrence's car and were on the road for ten days. There is no record of the car's reliability or where they stayed each night or how Lawrence managed his diet. The roads in northern France would still have been in a very poor state of repair after the destruction of the War. Another difficulty was that his chauffeur refused to drive through the busy streets of Paris, so Lawrence, in his debilitated state and with limited vision in one eye, took the wheel. When they reached England, the Italian refused to drive on the left, so once again Lawrence had to take over. They drove straight to King's, where Lawrence was admitted to the Casualty Ward in the evening of 28 May 1923, ten days after leaving Florence, 'more dead than alive, but no pre-coma, and the profound sleep was more from travel exhaustion than ketosis'. Dr Harrison greeted him, but it was decided to run various tests and delay the first dose of insulin for a few days so that the clinical effectiveness of the new drug could be assessed.

In a talk given at King's in 1961,[17] Lawrence said that he went to the laboratory as soon as it was open the following morning, 29 May 1923, at 10.30 am. His

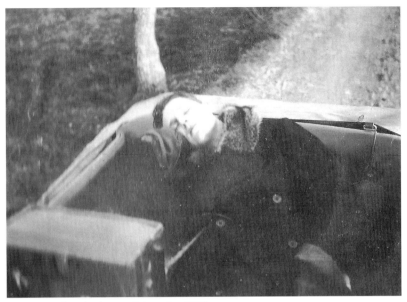

Lawrence asleep in the car, late spring 1923.

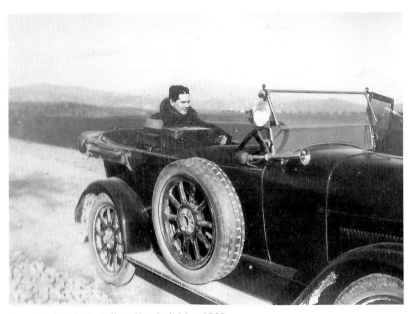

En route for King's College Hospital, May 1923.

blood sugar was found to be 410 mg per 100 ml (22.8 mmol/L); his urine was loaded with sugar (+++), and acetone bodies (++). Thereafter, he was tested every 90 minutes, the only major change relating to acetone, which increased to +++. The same procedure continued during 30 May. His weight was 9 stone 7 lb 9 oz, (60.55 kg, BMI 20 kg/m^2), which could not really be called wasted for a man of 5 ft

8 in (1.73 m) tall, but it was three stones less than in September 1917, when he was 12 stone 9 lb (80.29 kg).

On 31 May 1923, Dr Harrison 'went to the fridge, took out a bottle of insulin, and we discussed in our ignorance what the dose should be. It was all experimental, for I didn't know a thing about it; and neither did he for he had only treated about three people. So we decided to have 20 units – a nice round figure.'

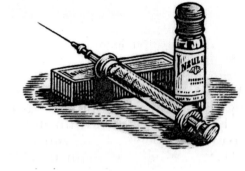

Insulin syringe.

The first dose was given at 10 am on 31 May, which Dr Harrison 'did so skilfully in my upper arm that I thought nothing of it compared with some horrid injections I had had of anti-tetanus, anti-plague, typhoid, and cholera – so I had no qualms about future insulin injections.' Lawrence then had breakfast of

Bacon and eggs and toast made on the Bunsen. I hadn't eaten bread for months and months, and I did this without feeling guilty. Hourly urine tests showed decreasing sugar and acetone until at 3 pm the urine was sugar-free. So we gave a cheer, not

Lawrence's own notes on his first dose of insulin.

a very loud one, for Banting and Best. But I didn't feel any different, neither better nor worse. However, at 4 pm, I had a terrible shaky feeling and a terrible sweat and an awful hunger pain. That was my first experience of hypoglycaemia (abnormally low blood sugar) However, we remembered that Banting and Best had described an overdose of insulin in their dogs. So I had some sugar and a biscuit or two, and soon got quite well, thank you.

This was the beginning of a remarkable personal and professional odyssey that would lead to Lawrence becoming the most famous diabetes specialist in Britain.

References

1. Harley G. *Diabetes: Its Various Forms and Different Treatments.* London, 1866.
2. Nothmann MM. The history of the discovery of pancreatic diabetes. *Bull Hist Med* 1954; **28**: 272–4.
3. Allen FM, Stillman E, Fitz R. *Total Dietary Regulation in the Treatment of Diabetes.* New York: The Rockefeller Institute for Medical Research, Monograph No.11,1919.
4. Williams JR. An evaluation of the Allen method of treatment of diabetes mellitus. *Am J Med Sci* 1921; **162**: 62–72.
5. Published as Harrison GA, Lawrence RD. Diastase in blood and urine as a measure of renal efficiency. *Lancet* 1923; **i**: 169–70.
6. Bliss M. *The Discovery of Insulin.* Chicago: University of Chicago Press, 1982.
7. Campbell WR. Anabasis. *Can Med Assoc J* 1962; **87**: 1055–61.
8. Banting FG, Best CH, Collip JB, et al. Pancreatic extracts in the treatment of diabetes mellitus: preliminary report. *Can Med Assoc J* 1922; **12**: 141–6.
9. The control of glycosuria by the islets of Langerhans. *Br Med J* 1922; **ii**: 140–1.
10. A full list of references to the British experience can be found in Tattersall RB. A force of magical activity: the introduction of insulin treatment in Britain 1922–1926. *Diabet Med* 1995; **12**: 739–55.
11. The part played by the MRC is described in more detail in Liebenau J. The MRC and the pharmaceutical industry: the model of insulin. In: Austoker J, Bryder L, eds. *Historical Perspectives on the Role of the MRC: Essays in the History of the Medical Research Council of the United Kingdom and its Predecessor, the Medical Research Committee 1913–1953.* Oxford: Oxford University Press, 1989: 163–80.
12. Macleod JJR. Insulin and diabetes. A general statement of the physiological and therapeutic effects of insulin. *Br Med J* 1922; **ii**: 833–7.
13. The treatment of diabetes by insulin. *Br Med J* 1922; **ii**: 991–2.
14. Banting FG, Campbell WR, Fletcher AA. Further clinical experience with insulin (pancreatic extracts) in the treatment of diabetes mellitus. *Br Med J* 1923; **i**: 8–12.
15. Insulin. *Br Med J* 1923; **i**: 341.
16. Insulin available in this country: conditions of sale and precautions to be observed. *Br Med J* 1923; **i**: 695–6.
17. Lawrence RD. Diabetes at King's. *KCH Gazette* 1961; **48**: 3.

CHAPTER 2

An Aberdeen Education

One detests Aberdeen with the detestation of a thwarted lover. It is the one haunting and exasperatingly lovable city in Scotland.

Lewis Grassic Gibbon[1]

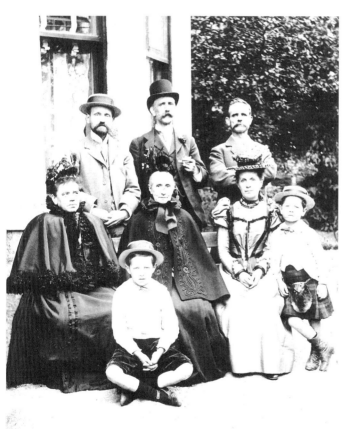

The Lawrence family gathered in all their finery c. 1897. Robin Lawrence strikes the one informal pose, leaning on his mother; he had an intensely close and loving relationship with her throughout her life. His father, Thomas Lawrence, is back left. Possibly 'Brushy' Morrison – Thomas's uncle – is back centre; Thomas's brother George is back right, without a hat. The widowed grandmothers are seated at the front: Grandmother Mary Smith on the left, Ann Lawrence in the centre. Young George is sitting cross-legged.

In the first part of this chapter about his childhood, R. D. Lawrence will be referred to as 'Robin', since there are so many references to the various Lawrences. In subsequent chapters, he will be referred to as 'Lawrence'.

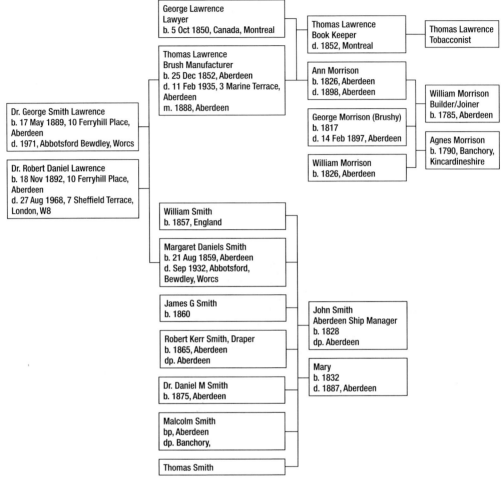

The Lawrence family tree.

Robin Lawrence's life began in Aberdeen, Scotland's third largest city, set between two rivers, the Don and the Dee. With its large granite buildings, it can appear grim under a gunmetal sky, but when the sun comes out, the mica chips in the stone make it glint and sparkle.

Robin's relations had lived in Aberdeen for several generations. His paternal great-grandfather Thomas was a tobacconist whose son, a bookkeeper also named Thomas, emigrated to the St Henri district of Montreal in 1849 and was later joined by his fiancé from Aberdeen, Ann Morrison. Thomas and Ann were married in September of the same year, and had their first son George in 1850. Ann's husband Thomas died in 1852 during her second pregnancy. She moved back to Aberdeen with George, who had barely turned two, and gave birth to her second son, Robin's father Thomas, on Christmas Day 1852. She moved in with her brother George, known affectionately as 'Brushy' as he owned George

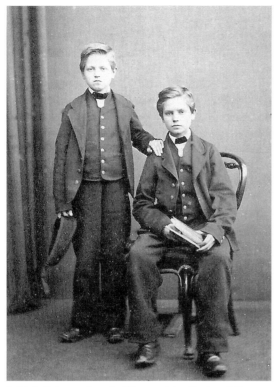

Robin's father and uncle: Thomas (standing) and George Lawrence wearing the uniform of Robert Gordon's Hospital, c. 1862.

Morrison & Co., brushmakers of 32 George Street Aberdeen. George was described in his obituary as 'a man of a quiet, reserved disposition … he never quite relinquished his old-fashioned ways; but was ever ready to do a kind action, and he was one of the most reliable of men.' His nephew Thomas Lawrence also developed many of these qualities.

Robin's father Thomas and his uncle George boarded at Robert Gordon's Hospital. To qualify for entry, boys had to be the sons or grandsons of a Burgess of Guild of the City of Aberdeen[2] who would not otherwise be able to afford to give them an education. The boys were educated free of charge and were also provided with a uniform with distinctive pelicans on the silver buttons. When they left the Hospital, the boys were apprenticed to a master, with the Governors paying their apprenticeship fees. At the end of their indenture, if they had performed well, the Governors awarded them £10 to set up in business for themselves. Robert Gordon's original aim was to fit poor boys for a trade. The school became a fee-paying day school and changed its name to Robert Gordon's College in 1881.

George and Thomas were taught English Reading, Grammar and Composition, Writing, Arithmetic, and Church Music, with the Outlines of History and Evidences of Christianity. In addition, to quote from the Statutes of 1850, 'Such of them as discover superior talents shall be taught all or any of the following branches, viz Book-keeping, French, Latin, the Elements of Geometry, Trigonometry, Navigation and Natural Philosophy, Geography and Drawing'. Both Thomas and George seized these educational opportunities. George went into a law firm, where he remained all his working life, and Thomas was apprenticed to Brushy Morrison's business in 1885 on his uncle's retirement. He ran the business successfully until his own retirement at 73 in 1924.[3] Victorian and early Edwardian households needed a vast array of brushes before the advent of mechanized cleaning. It was only from his obituary in the Aberdeen press in 1935 that the sons learned that their father Thomas had supplied all the brushes to Queen Victoria and her successors at Balmoral Castle. It was not something that Thomas chose to flaunt.

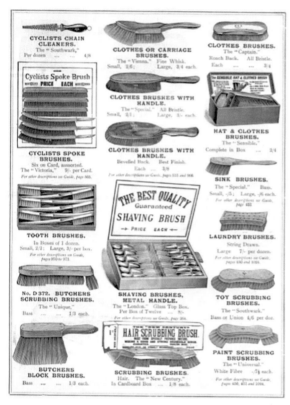

A large range of brushes was needed in the Victorian household (advertisement from a 1901 catalogue).

In the Lawrence family archive, there is a carefully preserved testimonial with the heading 'Aberdeen February 13th 1840':

I Hereby certify that Mr. John Lawrence Member of the Royal College of Surgeons in London was a most distinguished student at the Anatomy Class in Marischal College, that he performed many dissections of the human body, with the greatest care and that he was at such pains to acquire a sound knowledge of the various branches of medical science.

I had many communications with Mr. Lawrence and can safely say that I believe him to be well qualified for practising his profession.

The paper was signed by 'William Pirrie MD of Edinburgh. Surgeon Formerly Lecturer on Anatomy in the University of Aberdeen. Now Professor of Surgery at Marischal College.' It is not clear where this ancestor fits into the family tree, but Robin had a long held ambition to become a surgeon and it is possible that knowledge of this relative, a great uncle perhaps, had inspired that ambition.

In 1888, Thomas married Margaret Daniels Smith, daughter of the late John Smith, Manager of the London and Aberdeen Steamship Company. She had been brought up in the harbour area of Aberdeen, which for centuries was a thriving port as

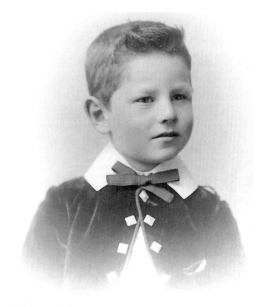

Robin aged 6.

well as a shipbuilding one. A year after their marriage, a son, George Smith Lawrence, was born on 17 May 1889 in the three-storied granite house at 10 Ferryhill Place, followed 2½ years later on 18 November 1892 by Robert Daniel, who emerged unscathed after a breech birth. We know about the birth from a letter from a university friend, who referred to Robin having entered life 'posterior priores'. It was a particularly cold winter, and the baptism, conducted by Professor Inverach, Professor of Apologetics at the University, took place at home over two months later – according to the baptismal records, this was quite unusual, as the vast majority took place in the church itself. It is possible that Maggie Lawrence was not well enough to attend any ceremony away from home.

Thomas Lawrence was described by Robin as 'a mild, modest parent whom I soon learned to dominate'. His photos show a calm face where no sign of emotion is betrayed, but perhaps that tells us more about the style of Victorian photography than the true nature of Thomas Lawrence. He was a serious man, an elder at Queen's Cross Church, a golfer, a bowls player and a keen supporter of the temperance movement. Thomas, an academic man whose chosen career would not have been in brushes, became a supportive, kind, generous and an admirably ambitious parent to his two sons. He was keen to further their talents in every way and, to this end, provided generously for them. He also had a lighter side to him, as Robin noted how enjoyable it was 'when motor cars were introduced, especially when my Father was racing my uncle.' Thomas managed the business successfully, but his real interest lay in books and the house was full of the novels of Walter Scott, Thackeray and Dickens, which Robin devoured when he learned to read. George was also an avid reader, and when they became young men, George's letters to Robin were full of literary references. Later, George named his Worcestershire home 'Abbotsford' after Scott's house in Melrose.

Robin described his mother as 'a sort of Christian angel, loved by all the neighbours as well as her own family'. From her portraits, she does seem to emanate a calm, angelic quality. Robin's older brother George had a similar disposition and Robin recalled that when he had ruined some of George's favourite toys, his mother asked George, 'Why don't you punish him?', but the mild George just replied, 'I can't smack Robin.' George, however, was no meek pushover. As a young man, he had a distinguished military record and was awarded the Military Cross during the First World War.

As a small boy, his mother called Robin her 'cockie doodle'. He was exceptionally close to her and throughout his three years in India during the First World War (Chapter 4) he was to write a steady stream of warm and loving letters to her. She had started him on scales on the piano, and then on Scottish melodies, laying the foundation of his great love of music. Later they enjoyed playing piano duets for four hands. Their family entertainment was held round the piano using Robin's well-worn copy of the *Scottish Students' Song Book*.

As a toddler, Robin's favourite walk was 'to our station, a small terminus where the engine driver friendly to children – or was it to Nanny's charms? – gave us a ride on his old puffing Billy as he did his shunting'. He developed and maintained a passion for steam trains throughout his life and in the 1950s wrote an article mourning the passing of the steam age.

Robin records joining George at Miss Downie's[4] school close by in Ferryhill, at the age of five, 'resplendent in a kilt (Gordon tartan, of course)', where he found the 'pretty little girls liked my kisses – or was it the kilt and sporran?' George transferred to Aberdeen Grammar School in 1897 and Robin joined him in August 1900, aged nearly eight. At the time, there were around 500 boys in the school. From extracts in the school magazine, one can see that Robin was a versatile and talented boy with academic, sporting and musical gifts who even managed to carry off a prize for 'Sword Feats on a Bicycle' in the annual school sports.

He studied Latin, Greek and French, for which he had quite a good accent. Rugby was the school game, and at every spare moment the boys would practise converting imaginary tries. Much later on, a Grammar School old pupils' team was formed '(the best in the N of Scotland)', and some of its members, including Robin, were asked to play in the Scottish Trials. Robin noted, 'One thing we learned at the Grammar School was how to work at books. I remember sons of rich and snobbish parents who had been sent to Public Schools who, having failed Matriculation, came back to the Grammar School at the age of 16 to study hard, like us. I found the Matriculation examination quite easy.'

At home on Sundays, the family went to morning worship at Queen's Cross Church, where his father was an Elder and Robin enjoyed singing hymns and psalms before snoozing against his mother's sealskin cape during the sermon and then skipping home to a dinner of roast Aberdeen Angus and a special pudding; his favourite was roly poly. The family would relax briefly after their Sunday lunch chewing humbugs known as stripies and having a smoke before taking a turn round the hill. Robin was sent to Sunday school, where he enjoyed reading the Old Testament as he thought it 'rather fun', but he also had to learn the Catechism, which he did not understand and claimed he never would. After supper, to bed and prayers with his mother, which had a conventional start along the lines of 'God bless father, mother, Georgie, etc., and make me a good boy'. However, the young angler with his scientific mind went on with another prayer of his own: 'Dear God, high above the clouds and thus controlling them, please when I am going fishing send enough rain to keep the burns flowing gently, but not enough for a pea-soup flood.' But although he prayed this frequently and with fervour, 'Jupiter never controlled the rain clouds for me. So a spirit of agnosticism was born in me, the angler.'

Robin wrote that 'at that time in Presbyterian Scotland, religious instruction started very early, especially when the father was an Elder of the Kirk and the mother a devoted Christian as mine were'. It was at Sunday School of all places that he committed his first crime. The Superintendent was a fat pompous man, who wore a stiff white shirt with gold cuff links. One Sunday, while the Superintendent was waving and prattling nearby, one of his cuff links fell at Robin's feet. It flashed attractively and Robin picked it up and put it in his sporran pocket. He thought the Superintendent, and certainly the timid headmistress, would not think of looking there, but on his return home, his mother did and chastised him for his double

RUBISLAW DEN NORTH

crime of theft and lying. She resorted to the *wait-until-your-father-comes-home* approach, but Robin told her that it would be no use as his father was not strong enough or adequately fierce. He prescribed his own punishment – a strapping from his grandmother, who did the job so well that Robin decided never to lie or steal again.

In 1899, the Lawrence family moved to a larger house in Rubislaw Den North, which was considered the smartest area of Aberdeen. Robin wrote in his draft autobiography that 'there wasn't really an "East End" in Aberdeen except for a small area about the harbour where the trawler men, their wives and numerous children lived in slummery'. This move benefited the boys, as they were now able to bicycle to school, 'there being no dangerous traffic (and all downhill) in five minutes, and only some seven minutes home again, driven by an aching hunger, especially after rugger'.

He certainly came from a loving, comfortable, middle-class home, where he was presented with a great many opportunities, but he also put effort into his work, sport and music. The family went on local holidays to Torphins, Banchory, and Stonehaven. His parents would also visit various hydros to try

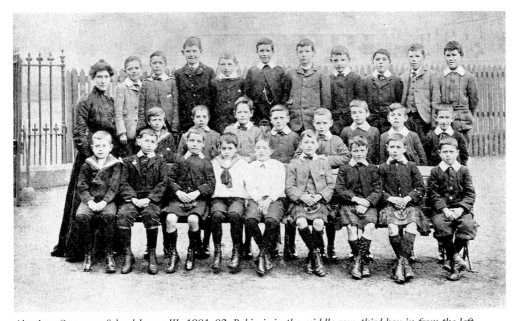

Aberdeen Grammar School Lower III, 1901–02. Robin is in the middle row, third boy in from the left.

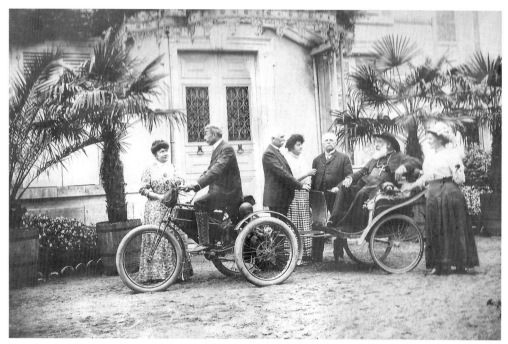

The family in Brittany, where Robin stayed in 1911 to learn French and possibly to enjoy a ride on this motorized tricycle with dogcart.

to bring about some relief for Maggie Lawrence's asthma. There were trips to the seaside and they often went up Deeside on the train, stopping off to visit the Falls of Feugh on their way to Ballater. Robin had fond memories of his mother's Deeside picnic parties. In winter, he skated on the boating pond at Duthie Park and developed a lifelong love of the activity. They also travelled to the Loire and to Switzerland for a family holiday, which was quite unusual at that time. Robin spent some time living with a family in Brittany to learn French.

Very early in his life he developed a passion for fishing, and in his autobiographical notes there are many sketches of his fishing exploits. He had the sharpest eye for detail, for small signs and indications of the possible whereabouts of the fish. He contributed to the smooth running of the home and became chief weeder of the gooseberry patch. When he went on fishing expeditions, he would raid the garden compost heap for a good supply of worms, which he kept in moss and oatmeal before using them as bait. During the early part of the Second World War, he worked with earthworms again and cleaned them in the way he learned in his childhood. He and his wartime collaborator then analysed the protein content of the worms with a view to their use in supplementing the nation's diet during the war.[5]

There are few other mentions of his childhood in the autobiographical notes he made towards the end of his life. He merely summed it up by saying that early life was very kind to him.

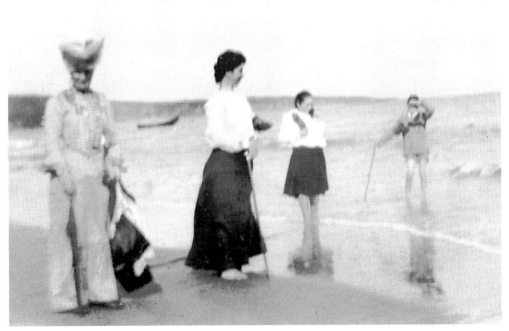

Three generations on Aberdeen beach, Robin paddling.

Robin became particularly aware of just how charmed his early life in Aberdeen had been when he went to visit relations:

It wasn't until I paid a visit to my Uncle Daniel in Liscard near Birkenhead that I learned that the entire world was not as friendly as it was at home. His house was very near the Mersey, and after breakfast I used to go down to what was called 'the beach' to dig and build sand castles. No doubt I made disparaging remarks about the dirty oily sand in comparison with the clean sand of Aberdeen, and my unknown dress (the kilt) must have aroused the ire and curiosity of the English boys. One day I was surrounded by some ten hostile young boys. Who started the attack I don't remember, but soon there was blood flowing from Liverpudlian noses. They disappeared and left me in triumph. My doctor uncle received many complaints from irate parents, but he took my side and his only answer, if any, was – 'Ten to one, disgraceful!' After this I greatly enjoyed going round on his visits in a smart cabriolet drawn by a spanking piebald. My only complaint was that he didn't come out with shillings or even pennies which I thought he might have given me. My pocket money was one penny a week, but I soon discovered a sweet-shop where I got far more of my liquorice strips than in Aberdeen.

Robin's maternal Uncle Robert (Bob) was a draper who married later in life and went on to have three children: Malcolm, May and Sheila. Before his marriage, Robert lived with the Lawrence family on the top floor, where there was a bedroom and a smoking room, large enough for a three-quarter size billiard table. Robin soon learned to beat his father at billiards as his father only enjoyed golf and bowling, but Uncle Bob was a different matter – he had a good eye and touch. He taught Robin useful skills such as 'side' and screwing back, which made him nearly an unbeatable opponent in his adult life. The only time Robin notched up a win against his uncle was the time cigar smoke began to get into Bob's eyes.

At the end of his time at the Grammar School, Uncle Bob shrewdly pointed out to Robin that if he went into Medicine, even on a professor's salary he would not be able to afford to rent a good salmon beat on the Dee. It was suggested that instead he become an apprentice draper in Edinburgh or Glasgow before returning to Aberdeen. He would be able to fish or play sport at the weekend. The financial advantages seemed attractive and so began Robin's short career as an apprentice draper. One Saturday when he was in charge of the shop, a handsome lady in a fur coat came in leading a small boy whom she wanted fitted out with warm underwear. Once this had been done, Robin remembered that the day before a charming collection of silk underpants had been delivered and asked the mother if she would like to be the first to see them. He blustered along in his sales pitch with great confidence, giving an excellent impression to his customers of being on top of the situation and remembered the scene as follows:

'Oh, they're lovely: they are not pants but knickers' – a new word for me. 'They are not very warm, but are for beauty and attraction.' (Good: I've learned something!) 'Have you anything else to show me?' I had indeed, but I remembered my position, and suggested a pair of black silk stockings, a contrast to lead up to the exciting pink knickers! 'Will you have the things sent on or pay and take them with you', I asked. 'I'll take them', she said: so I added up the bill and asked for 'Five Guineas please.'

The following Monday the boss greeted me with, 'I have to congratulate you on your salesmanship last Saturday. You not only got warm underclothes for the child, but actually sold knickers and stockings which the lady didn't come for – and she paid cash. I have been thinking of promoting you to the glove department and now this has decided me.' 'Thank you', I said. 'I'm sure my uncle will be pleased. But, excuse me; I have decided that to be a rich draper is not the life for me, although I have been happy here with all your kindness. I shall return to Aberdeen to study medicine and become a doctor like my family before.'

Medical school

Aberdeen University was founded in 1495 in Old Aberdeen to the north of the modern city centre. Robin's move from the Grammar School to King's College at the University in 1909 was almost seamless. He could still live at home; his brother George was already studying there and many contemporaries from school went with him to enter the University as bajans, the curious name given to first-year

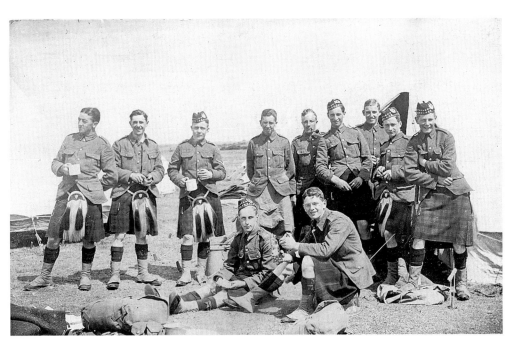

From Robin's album: Territorial Company of the 3rd Gordon Highlanders (Grammar School 1909). Robin is in the back row, right-hand end – without a sporran. He found it too uncomfortable for walking and was punished for this and had to clean out the 'dixie' in which the breakfast kippers had been cooked. He noted 'all those other Gordon Highlander territorials were killed in 1914' and he kept the photograph on his desk throughout his life.

medical students, as well as others in the Gordon Highlanders from school cadet camps.

On the sporting front, he gave up rugger and changed to hockey and he also joined the tennis team. Robin, with his capacity for hard work coupled with his formidable memory, had a very successful first year, for he was awarded Class 1 and was a prizeman in both examinations. His family was delighted with his success and for his 18th birthday his father gave him a baby Bechstein grand piano, which in today's money is roughly equivalent to being given a top-of-the-range car.

It was common for students at Aberdeen to start with an Arts course. Lectures were compulsory, with a roll call being taken at the beginning of each session. Robin's brother George had entered the university in 1907 to study Latin, English, German and Moral Philosophy, before switching to Medicine in 1912. Robin chose to take an MA in English under 'a most stimulating professor' and French 'under an Alsatian, whose accent would not have been approved of at Grammar School.' He also studied French and Zoology, but then registered in April 1910 as a medical student at Marischal College, which was then part of the unified University of Aberdeen.

Robin's first-year medical studies did not thrill him; he was awarded a 2nd Class Certificate in Systematic Chemistry and a 1st Class one in Osteology. Living in the far northeast, he had long hours of daylight to help him to learn the names of the 200 bones in the human body well into the night, but his family suffered during that summer term, for when darkness eventually fell and he could no longer see the list of bones, he would go into the well-lit music room to play Beethoven sonatas on the piano around midnight. When examined in osteology, he had to watch his manners:

I knew osteology fairly well except for a few such stupid questions on which my brain refused to waste mental energy, e.g. 'Here is a small wrist bone – how would you distinguish between right and left?' 'I'm afraid I can't', and I longed to add 'Why do you ask such a silly question?', but always remembered that it didn't pay to cheek an examiner.

His next course involved the dissecting room, where he thought he had been given the best corpse to work on. Robin described him as 'a lean old man, a handsome fellow, who must have been a failure in life as he came from the poor house as did most of the corpses in the medical school', but he wished the old chap could have known what a vital role he'd played in stimulating his interest. Robin would get to the dissecting room as early as possible to prevent any other student interfering with what he described in his draft autobiography as my 'old pet's body'. It was the dissecting room that completely changed his life by introducing reality into his studies. Dissection went on until noon, when the students went to a demonstration by a particularly dull old professor of anatomy, Robert Reid (1851–1939), who could barely maintain his students' interest, but they kept alert by counting the number of times he scratched his nose with an alarmingly dirty finger. Robin felt that Reid was only at home in the depths of the chilly dissecting room with its all-pervasive odour of formalin, but he is remembered today for having founded the University Anthropological Museum.

After a good wash, the medics lunched in the Students' Union, where Robin's usual fare was a glass of milk and all the bread and butter with an occasional scrape of jam that a penny would buy. This was followed by a game of billiards before going to the Physiology Department, where he found an inspiring teacher in the professor, John Alexander MacWilliam FRS (1857–1937), a pioneer in cardiac electrophysiology who elucidated the mechanism of sudden cardiac death from ventricular fibrillation and who was years ahead of his time in suggesting it could be reversed by an electric shock. At the end of the academic year 1911–12, Robin was awarded a handsomely bound copy tooled with gold of Osler's famous textbook *The Principles and Practice of Medicine*. It was for the highest distinction in the senior division of the Anatomy Class.

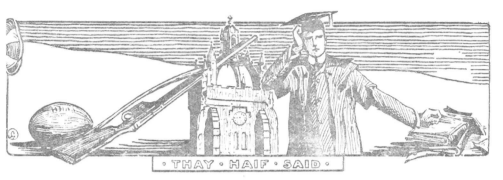

Masthead from the Alma Mater.

It is from old copies of the *Alma Mater*, the Aberdeen University student magazine, that we can learn so much else of this period in Robin's life. By 1911, it was a flourishing weekly publication with a leader or two on current questions and a miscellany of serious, informative, newsy and gossipy articles full of in-house student humour. There were cartoons, photographs and advertisements, including weekly ones from both the Rotunda and Coombe Hospitals in Dublin, urging students to enlist for their Obstetrics course. The Rotunda's advert boasted that over 4000 births took place each year, which would enable a student to achieve the requisite number of deliveries (20) in a very few weeks.

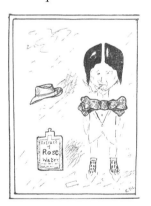

Cartoons by Jack Mason (right) and Robin in the Alma Mater, *20 December 1911. Mason has depicted Robin, and his caption reads 'Cynical smile of my dearest friend (or anyone else) admiring my cartoon.' The subject of Robin's cartoon is obscure; it might relate to his friend G. W Rose, but it certainly shows his early fancy for bow ties.*

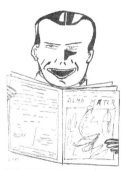

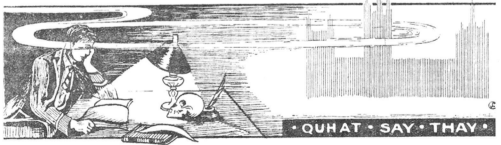

With a gun apparently to his head in the masthead and a skull to stare up at him in the lower one, student life around the turn of the 20th century could appear quite stressful.

In a world without radio or television, there were fewer distractions in the lives of students and Friday afternoon had yet to be regarded as a time for winding down.[6] These university societies met on Friday afternoons at staggered times so that individuals could attend more than one, and their agenda was packed with serious topics. Robin was elected to the Medical Society in 1911 and made his maiden speech that November with 'an able address' on 'Hypnosis and its Value as a Therapeutical Agent'. His audience was described as 'interested, but half sceptical.' He concentrated on its uses in the treatment of functional rather than organic disorders and gave 'instances in which it had proved eminently successful'. His paper was 'keenly discussed' and he described a case where a chronic constipation was cured when all drugs had failed. In later years, Robin was wary of anything that even hinted at fringe medicine and it is slightly surprising that he chose this subject for his maiden speech. In the following month, Robin and the committee of the Medical Society organized a presentation on 'Salvarsan and Syphilis.' Salvarsan was an arsenic-based treatment for syphilis, which appeared in 1910 and was heralded as a miracle cure. The magazine report of the meeting noted 'the lecturer first dealt with the history of Syphilis – with its introduction into, and rapid growth on, the virgin soil of Europe'.

He made his debut in the Literary Society with a paper on the life and works of W. S. Gilbert, including the partnership with Sir Arthur Sullivan.

Robin was elected to the committee of the *Alma Mater* in 1911 when his friend and near neighbour Jack Mason was editor. They had much in common and were described as being full of life and *joie de vivre* and as having a wide variety of interests and accomplishments. Both were charming men with magnetic personalities. They were very well read and talented musicians. They worked together on the magazine for two years with Robin's friend from the tennis team, Walter Inkster, who contributed most of the cartoons. Mason's term of office as Editor with Robin as Assistant Editor was described later in the *Alma Mater* as a bright one in the history of the magazine.

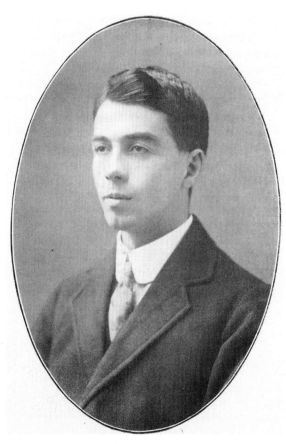

Lawrence's close friend JHS Mason who was editor of the Alma Mater 1911–1912

Robin played tennis and hockey regularly and was unlucky not to have been awarded a tennis blue in the match versus Edinburgh. The report for the 1910–11 season tells us that he 'plays a fairly consistent game; was reserve man for the first six and had the pleasure of playing against Edinburgh 'Varsity when he and his partner had very hard lines in not getting a match. He ought to be very good next season.'

Robin's university life from 1909 to 1912 was packed not only with his wide spread of subjects – Anatomy, Chemistry, Natural Philosophy, Embryology, Botany, Physiology, Materia Medica and Political Economics – but was also with the production of the weekly edition of *Alma Mater*. By December 1912, he was on the Committee for the Medicine Class Supper with his friends Robert Boulton-Myles and Tom Menzies. Robin replied to the toast 'The World and his Wife' and also played a Spanish Fantasy on the piano, neither of which could have been easy after the feast of hare soup, boiled halibut, chicken patties, roast saddle of mutton, roast turkey, plum pudding and wine jelly.

In July 1912, he went to stay in Rostock, an old Hanseatic town in northern Germany. The purpose of the visit was to learn German, attend some medical lectures, relax, read and play the piano seriously. At one time, he had even thought of devoting his career to music.

He kept a diary throughout this period and wrote many letters home. Both diary and letters reveal a gentle pace of life more suited to an elderly convalescent than

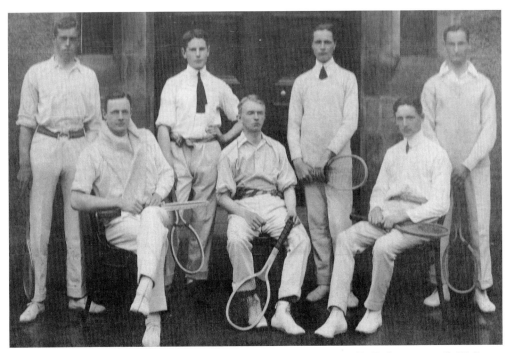

Aberdeen University Tennis Club, 1910–11. Standing (L to R): J. I. Watson, **R. D. Lawrence**, *C. W. Rose (a triple blue, RAMC, killed in action 1917). Seated (L to R): F. F. Brown, C. A. Laing, W. Inkster. (From Robin's photograph collection.)*

an energetic young blade from medical school. He drank a great deal of milk as he had discovered that coffee kept him awake, talked much of afternoon snoozes (and sometimes morning ones as well) and enjoyed the comfort of nursery puddings.

He read the Life of Beethoven, which prompted him to note that he could now understand the composer's music better. He also tackled Schiller, Goethe, and a Life of Wagner. He attended a few lectures at the University of Rostock on Physiology and also on Anatomy. The halting and somewhat dutiful letter sent to his aunt and uncle in Aberdeen captures the tone of his visit:

It is now close on nine o'clock and I have finished my supper and lit my lamp and I am sitting on a sofa, but it is not an English one. It is uncomfortable and is so high that I write at the table as well as I could from a chair. I have been meaning for some time to write, and at last I have got to begin. It is dark now, the sky is dull and it even rains a little. I hope you are having really satisfactory weather to please everyone (except the farmers of course). I can imagine you all after dinner, sitting, reading or sewing, chatting and eating 'stripies', perhaps smoking a cigarette, but you are not German ladies and perhaps don't smoke. In Rostock, some smoke, not many, however and not ladies of such a status as yours. In Warnemünde [a seaside

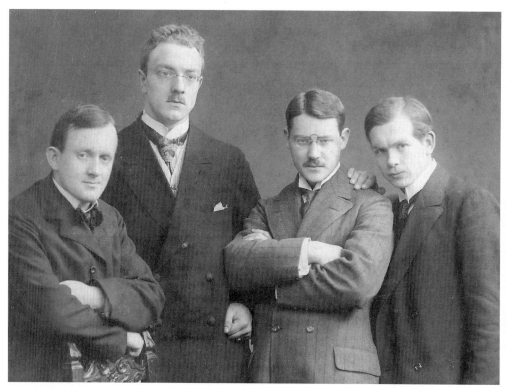

Robin, second in from right, aged 19, with his friends from Rostock in Germany – a serious set of young students who enjoyed working, talking and music making together and who would soon be at war against each other.

*town near Rostock], the after-meal cigarette is very common and between meals too
for women, old and young alike. I am smoking about once a week, so not too much.*

*The days slip round now very quickly, and all much in the same fashion. Today
has been typical. In the morning, I went at nine to my German teacher and put
in a very profitable hour with him. He is very particular about pronunciation and
if my German pronunciation is not very good, I could at least know when anyone
talks good German. I should be interested to hear George read when I come home.
Huhnhauser (teacher) is very careful about the niceties of pronunciation. I do
dictation, reading and translation in a crowded hour, or rather, I often get an extra
quarter of an hour. After the lesson we generally adjourn to the piano and I play his
accompaniments. He is a magnificent singer and was trained for it for four years:
then, however, he became a teacher. Unfortunately he has no soft notes in his reach.
It is either* pp, f. or ff. *We have been doing Schubert songs and Schumann's.*

*I then come home to drink a glass of milk somewhere and rest while on a seat
in some public place. At 11.30 go to Frau Fick and read German for half an hour
with her and then English for as long again. Fortunately, I get more German out
of it than she English. We are always speaking German. Her pronunciation is
atrocious, and when I correct it she cannot always pronounce English correctly
even then.*

*Today, I ate with the Ficks, but usually I stroll to my pension to eat with the silent
Germans. They eat very fast and have very strange sauces, which I must avoid for
my stomach's sake. After dinner, I come home and sleep a bit.*

*Then today I went out at 3.30 to play tennis again with the Ficks. I came home
about seven after a very pleasant afternoon and set to getting supper ready. I have a
spirit lamp and cooked two eggs on it. I buy in breakfast; butter, marmalade and of
these I make my meal. Frau Prop supplies milk and cleans the pan. For a change I
have cheese, ham or veal or go to a restaurant I have discovered. Usually my supper
costs me about six or seven pfennig, and I am quite satisfied with that.*

*So now you know pretty well how my days roll by, and it will only be necessary in
the future to describe any excursions or special events.*

He sent home a stream of such letters to friends and relations detailing the
minutiae of his life, and he received many in return. His young friends from
Aberdeen were away on similar trips. They were a literary bunch with serious tastes
in art and architecture. One particular lady friend, Nellie Conner, proudly noted
that she had visited six chateaux in one day on her tour of the Loire.

Robin's father wrote asking him to notice and assess everything he saw. He kept a
list in the back of his diary of all the areas in which he should glean the information
that his father thought so important: students, workmen, shopmen, women, boys,
children, town, streets, post, food, drink, clothes, exercise, education and theatre.
At one point, he wondered if he'd be taken for a spy. He notes the fondness the
local students have for smoking:

*more than do most of our students, the proportion being perhaps 40 cigarettes a day
instead of 14–20, and 10–12 cigars in place of 4–5 pipes. In summer at least, they
must average about 8 glasses of beer a day – far too much. Many of the students are*

already very fat, though they are still young; while it is almost impossible to find a German of 40–50 who is not more or less round and full-necked.

In another letter, he mentions lectures and a practical:

18th July 1912 … I went with Reid to a surgery clinic just to see how they were conducted. It was from 9–10 and immediately afterwards the cases who have been examined in the clinic are operated on by the surgeon and assistants. The surgery struck me as very poor. I should not care to have an operation under Dr. Müller and still less from his assistants. Either the standards here must be very low or else Aberdeen very high.

The students here work under quite a different system from ours. They have two examinations: the first includes our first and second professionals; the second, our 3rd and final. The first is at the end of their 3rd year and the second at the fifth. Between these times, they have no examinations, no class examinations, no sign-ups, no attendances to put in at classes (for there is no attendance roll and attendance is quite voluntary). So, as a rule, they do nothing for their first year and a half perhaps two years, and then do a burst of work to get through. They slack off again during the fourth year. The one limit that is set to enjoyment is lack of money.

Brother George wrote regularly and his letters are thoughtful and serious. He was very keen to guide Robin's reading:

What have you started to read? Don't let your man palm off any cheap stuff on you in the way of novels. Try and get some Otto Ernst's comedies if you can; they are colloquial and very funny. Seial, Kingelgen, Rosegger, Auerbach in small quantities are all good German … get your man to run over as much as possible for your own pleasure.

George passes on the concerns of their mother, saying that

Mother entreats you to be very prudent in your movements around Rostock in case you are caught up and clapped into prison for looking at the smoke of a German submarine. … The best befall thee, dear brother, with love from all your own people. Your affectionate George.

Robin's reply to this letter passes on reassurance to his mother about Anglo-German relations, and notes that the Germans feel quite friendly towards the English. He tells George that he's reading a book about Wagner, whom the Germans hold in the highest regard:

However, it's getting late and I must always to bed early for the nerves. Vita Placida. *I reserve my judgment on German girls till I know some. They are not pretty up here in the North. Much love Georgie from your brother.*

He had several musical sessions with friends and went to the opera to hear Wagner's *The Flying Dutchman*:

A funny play, didn't impress or stir me. Opera is a queer mixture, music, singing words, acting and scenery. For me so many simultaneous mediums of expression are confusing. Orchestra of about 100. V Strauss leading. The actors sometimes made gestures in keeping with the music and walked in time with it etc. Even when they were not singing. I didn't like that. Why? It made it seem as if they were thinking with the orchestra, that the music was their very thoughts, translated word by word into phrase by phrase of theme and variation. No time to think. Actresses a bit fat, but fine singers and mostly quiet actors. The Flugende Hollander *has perhaps too many small crises. I was somewhat too near to appreciate the music at its best.*

Opera never found a place in his heart, although he later enjoyed the works of Puccini and Verdi. He went to several concerts in his six weeks at Rostock, including one with 'beautiful German songs amongst other "Rose Garten" and "Untren". The Rostock male voice choir gave old songs and ballads and between times we had Wagner and Cherubini from an orchestra. Beer and pipe at the same time.'

Robin did a great deal of piano playing during his time in Rostock. He played some Beethoven duets 'very badly' with a friend, and tried some Schubert, which was 'very pleasing'. He accompanied a Mozart violin sonata for a friend – 'too much of the Haydn'. He spent much time listening to Beethoven's symphonies: '... 6th 9th and 7th. The 3rd is glorious. It is impossible to decide which I like most; they are so wonderfully varied in mood and matter.'

On the eve of his departure from Rostock, he had a farewell dinner of epic proportions with friends where he was presented with a fine copy of Beethoven's Letters. They ate, drank, sat on the sofas talking and laughing before one friend sang a song. Robin then played two Beethoven sonatas: *Das Lebewohl* and the *Appassionata*, which must have been quite a feat after such an evening.

In one letter, he described the Kaiser:

Seems well liked. Huhnhauser said he was popular. Far more postcards of him and in the Royal House are for sale in the shops than of King George. Or perhaps, Aberdeen is not a loyal place. Reid did not like him for the reason that he is too outspoken. Kaiser is King of Prussia and leader of the German Army and Navy. He is head of both when war breaks out, though I expect, more a nominal than a real head. Each kingdom has its own Großherzog *(Grand Duke) who is much what the Kaiser is in Prussia.*

His parents systematically circulated every letter to the aunts and uncles during his absence, and his friends and family anticipated his return eagerly. One from Aberdeen ended his fond letter: 'What's this dull town to me, Robin's no there?' Robin returned to university in Aberdeen in the autumn of 1912 at a time when the Germany of Beethoven, Schiller and Goethe that he so appreciated was soon to be overtaken by the Kaiser, Prussia and militarism.

Back in Aberdeen, his teachers suggested that he try the primary FRCS examination. In London, he was met by an uncle and stayed overnight in his flat. Next morning, after a good breakfast, he went to meet his examiners at the Royal College of Surgeons:

Both were charming old surgeons – old enough I thought to have forgotten their general Anatomy except for the parts they operated on. So I answered their questions as briefly and to the point as I could, and was gratified to see them nodding consent to one another. Finally, one set a poser: 'What do you know of the balancing mechanism of the inner ear?' I answered 'Please give me a piece of chalk and I'll draw it on the blackboard.' While I was doing so, I saw him looking up the part concerned in his Anatomy book. 'Good, my boy: correct and clear: I think he deserves to pass the Anatomy most certainly and let us wish him success in Physiology.' This I enjoyed much more. They were younger professors, and told me some new facts in research which had not yet reached Aberdeen. They passed me too.

Robin returned to Aberdeen delighted with the results of his visit: 'In the train back north I looked upon myself as a mental hero. No second year medical student had ever passed this examination from Aberdeen. Whether I became a surgeon or not, I determined to keep up the highest standard of work that I could.' He certainly seems to have been regarded as a hero by his fellow students, as we shall hear in the next chapter.

References

1. Grassic Gibbon L. Aberdeen. In: *A Scots Hairst: Essays and Short Stories*. London: Hutchinson, 1967: 95–107 (originally published in Grassic Gibbon L, MacDiarmid H. *Scottish Scene: Or, The Intelligent Man's Guide to Albyn*. London: Jarrolds, 1934).
2. In 1222, a charter granted by Alexander II gave to the Burgh of Aberdeen the right to establish a Merchant Guild. Every merchant was obliged to join the Guild and only the Burgesses could sell their wares within the Burgh. On admission to the Guild, a trader made a contribution to its charitable funds, which were used to assist those Burgesses in need of financial help.
3. From his obituary in 1935 in an Aberdeen newspaper.
4. Aberdeen Grammar School records.
5. Lawrence RD, Millar HR. Protein content of earthworms. *Nature* 1945; **155**: 517.
6. McConachie J. *The Student Soldiers*. Elgin: Moravian Press, 1995. (This is the story of the Aberdeen University Company of the 4th Battalion of the Gordon Highlanders.)

CHAPTER 3

War Experiences of the Aberdonian Clan: 1914–1916

It was as if the spring had been taken from the year.

Pericles, when the youth of Athens had been destroyed in a terrible war[1]

These young students are cavorting on Aberdeen Beach in the summer of 1913 and the photographs mark the end of an era. The young men and the elegant bathing machines will soon be disappearing from British beaches. The photographs show the central role Lawrence played in his group of friends from the University. There is nothing of the hobbledehoy in him. He strikes poses; dainty pointed foot in one and rakish angle of the tam o' shanter in the other. He's the jaunty lad, the joker, and also the one who holds a key place in the group – as the following letters will reveal. The second photograph shows them taking a

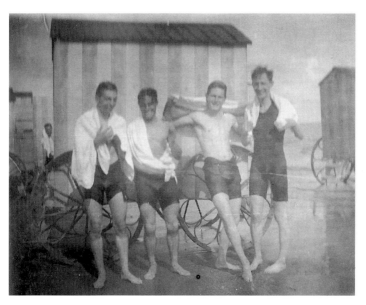

Aberdeen Beach, 1913. Lawrence is pointing his foot. Fifty years later, in a wavering hand, he entered the caption 'damned cold' in his album under this photograph.

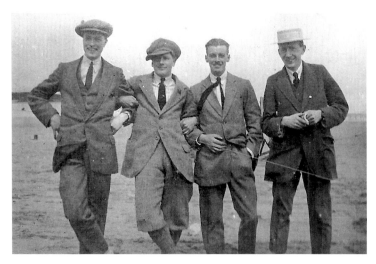

Aberdeen Beach, 1913. Lawrence is second from the left, with Boulton-Myles (left), Tom Menzies (?) and Robert Forgan.

break from their classes wearing their three-piece suits and probably spoiling their leather shoes with a rime of salt. They had recently returned from the first of their Officers' Training Camps at Aldershot.

After his successful trip to London for the primary FRCS examination in 1913, an open letter addressed to Lawrence in the *Alma Mater* issue of 11 February 1914 printed the sort of end-of-term report that a student can only dream of. Even the writer had to issue a warning: 'probably you are the best man of your year; certainly you are regularly returned at the head of the SRC (senior common room) poll, and your list of prizes is as hefty as ever.' These included the Fife Jamieson and Lazars Gold Medals in Anatomy awarded in 1913.[2]

But a mere catalogue of his manifold activities gives one no idea of the personal qualities of the man himself. Here we tread on more dangerous ground, for it has been the custom of writers of appreciative articles such as this to spread the butter very thickly, indeed, so much so that readers are unable to swallow it all. In Robin's case (with the Presidential permission we have temporarily abandoned the unaccustomed 'Mr. Lawrence') it is manifestly possible however, to be complimentary without entering the realms of romance. He has represented the Varsity at both hockey and tennis, and has also found time for swimming, billiards, rugby, cricket, motorcycling, riding and 'soccer', and in addition to all this he is a most expert angler.

In matters military he has the experience of a veteran, having served as a private in the Gordon Highlanders and as a cadet in the Officers' Training Corps, and he is now an officer in the RAMC (Special Reserve)

The article went on to comment on his personal qualities of

a frank and open manner, which, combined with a belief in himself, makes others put their confidence in him. Self-reliant, independent to a degree, he is none the less one of the most companionable fellows one could ever wish to meet.

He is described as

the most energetic man alive, 'high-spirited and bubbling over with joie de vivre, but nevertheless often unconscionably serious. We have talked with him well into the small hours on the most varied of subjects, though religion, women and the 'will to power' have always been our favourite themes. Fortunately, he is blessed with a sense of humour which allows him to laugh at himself: and his dignity is not a thing which bothers him much, when it is convenient to forget about it.

This encomium was written not long after the formal declaration of war by Britain on 4 August 1914, a war that scarred Lawrence forever and killed many of his friends.

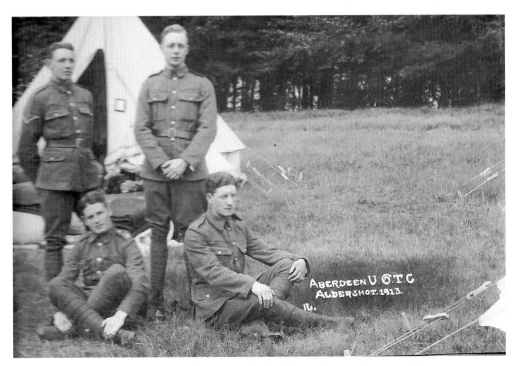

Lawrence seated front left at Aberdeen University Officers' Training Camp, Aldershot, 1913.

Lawrence's medical friends included Robert Forgan (1891–1976) known in the group as Ponto. He later became Executive Medical Officer to the Lanarkshire Joint Committee on Venereal Diseases and was Labour MP for West Renfrewshire. He was an able administrator and founder of the Medical Society for the Study of Venereal

Diseases (1922). He went on to play a key role in setting up Oswald Mosley's New Party. He organized work for the British Union of Fascists and became deputy leader; he resigned in 1934 when the Union began to campaign against Jews and after that took no active part in politics.

Another friend was Arthur (later Sir Arthur) Landsborough Thomson (1890–1977), known as Landsb, a distinguished medical administrator, mountaineer and ornithologist who pioneered Britain's first technique of ringing of birds when he was a student in 1909. Aged only 20, Thomson was elected to the British Ornithologists' Union.[3] John Ross MacNeill (1889–1956) became a surgeon. Tom (later Major-General) Menzies (1893–1969) was to specialize in tropical medicine and Robert Boulton-Myles (1893–1972) became a consultant radiologist. They called themselves the G.A.M.E. set, but the significance of this is not known. Forgan remained a lifelong friend with Lawrence, and Landsborough Thomson became very closely involved in Lawrence's later professional life.

A non-medical friend was Victor C. Macrae (known as Charlie), who with Lawrence shared a passion for fishing. There was Cecil Mackie and others too from his immediate neighbourhood; John Hampton Strachan Mason, known as Jack, from nearby Beaconsfield Place was reading English, followed a little later by a family friend from 16 Rubislaw Den, George Milne, and another friend called George Reid.

Charlie Macrae was described by his Professor as a 'strikingly able student' who gained his First-Class honours degree in classics after only a year's study. Despite his range of talents, Charlie was full of self-doubts and gained much confidence from Lawrence's company. He wrote from Rothesay in April 1914 telling him that the girls there had what he had heard called 'RSVP eyes' but that he had refrained

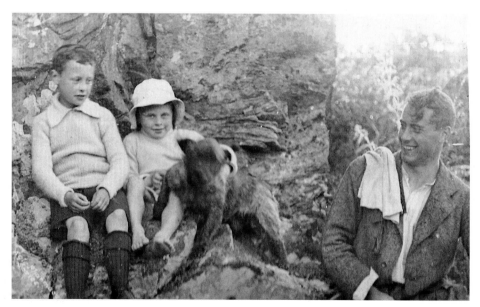

Victor Charles Macrae (Charlie) with young friends.

'almost entirely'. In a letter at the end of August 1914, Charlie confided that he had always been something of a 'mugwump' (an uncommitted person) as he did not know 'half the people I ought to owing to some mixture of shyness and laziness and lack of interest in me'. He continued:

You must make a psychological investigation some day into the case of the pleasure your letters afford me. They always indirectly put me in good spirits with myself, though how exactly I can't explain. I think there must be a subtle affinity between our attitudes to the world. I am always keenly conscious of mine towards it, so as I am marooned mentally when I am here, your epistles lay the spectre of self distrust which is apt to stalk whenever work or health goes wrong and the black butterflies begin to settle.

Charlie's letter continues in a tortuous and self-analytical way before telling Lawrence about an expedition where he had stalked cormorants and wild geese. He then settles on the topic of books he had read and ones that Lawrence might also like to read. He wishes him well with his continuing medical studies, 'Good hunting to yourself among the strange and manifold ruptures, tumours, wens, polypi and suppurations generally. I like hearing about them.'

In the spring of 1914 Lawrence was recovering from an appendectomy. It is probably that his appendix had burst, and over the next two years he was to have five or six laparotomies followed by a period of convalescence. In those pre-antibiotic days, the operation was needed to clear the pockets of pus that were left hiding in the abdomen. His abdominal wall was covered with multiple longitudinal scars and for the rest of his life he needed to wear a broad belt when exercising.

An Aberdonian medical colleague, (Alexander) Elmslie Campbell, was about to sail for Australia on the SS *Marathon* via Durban with the D'Oyly Carte Opera Company. He wrote in May 1914 to Lawrence and talked of arrangements for Lawrence to take over his work on a ward, and he urged him to do some reading on Surgery:

Appendicitis waits for no man ... you should now be on the high road to recovery and for a few weeks at least you trade on your convalescence to excite the every ready sympathy of some of your friends. As a pale faced convalescent, I guess you should be rather effective.

He wrote again to 'Dearest Robin' in July 1914 on his way back from Australia, where he had had a most interesting time and suggested that they both go out to the colonies at some time. He looked forward to his return on 3 September, by which time war had been declared.

From John McConachie's book *The Student Soldiers*,[4] we know that when war was declared, the 4th Territorial Battalion of the Gordon Highlanders was mobilized immediately at Aberdeen and with it the University Company, which formed about one-sixth of the battalion. Lawrence's friends Charlie Macrae, Cecil Davidson, George Reid, Stewart Paterson, Jack Mason and George Milne went either straight into active service or to Bedford for further training. Another friend, Walter Inkster – the apt name for a witty and talented cartoonist whose sketches had enlivened the *Alma Mater* for a year, returned from Australia to join the 4th Gordons with Jack Mason near Ypres. The medical students such as Lawrence whose studies were unfinished were encouraged to stay on at university. In 1915–16 this official encouragement applied only to the final-year students and conscription was introduced in 1916. It was not until 1915 that Lawrence's fellow medical students were mobilized. Lawrence's recurring bouts of illness prevented him from mobilizing and from sitting his exams.

There had been an Aberdeen University Company of the Gordon Highlanders long before the First World War. As John McConachie writes:

> It was a very popular and rewarding experience for many students – not unlike being a member of the football, shinty or rugby teams except that one volunteered to join rather than being chosen. There was also the small matter of pay. Students in those days were as impecunious as they are now, and Alma Mater was able to announce in October 1913 that the Company meeting would be held on 24th at Marischal College when arrears of pay would be distributed and promotions announced. It was hoped that every man would bring along his younger comrades to sign on as members of the best organisation in the Varsity. A keen first or second year student recruit, particularly one who excelled at some sporting activity, had every chance of promotion to the rank of non-commissioned officer.

Lawrence had been a cadet in the Gordon Highlanders at the Grammar School and had gone to training camp in the summer of 1909 and to an Officers' Training Camp at Aldershot in 1913. In July 1914, he became an officer in the RAMC

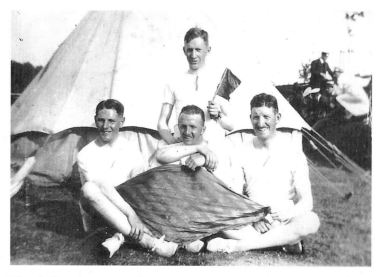

The winning relay team at the OTC Sports, Aldershot, 1914. Lawrence is front left. Robert Forgan (back) ran the final lap. He was a talented sportsman who had been capped for Scotland at hockey.

(Special Reserve) and went back to Aldershot with his fellow medical students Robert Boulton-Myles, Tom Menzies and Robert Forgan for further training. Lawrence thoroughly enjoyed this, especially tennis at the swell Officers' Club and learning to ride in the Hussars' riding school. He recalled that only farmers and their boys rode in Aberdeenshire and it took him a long time to do what the instructor wanted. This involved running beside his horse and jumping into the saddle without using the stirrups. He loved riding through the beautiful heather lanes, but on one occasion his horse suddenly shied and Lawrence took a tremendous toss, but fortunately landed on his bottom. 'I know not how I broke nothing except some wind, the noise of which seemed to scare the horse still more. He set off at a spanking trot down a side lane where I had great difficulty in catching him.'

Jack Mason, Charlie Macrae and George Milne went to summer training camp for U Company at Tain in 1914. One of the attractions of U Company was

> *The opportunity for wearing the kilt and the striking sporran which were provided free with the rest of the uniform. In those days of predominantly dark and somewhat drab clothes the student soldiers would have cut quite a dash – particularly in female eyes – and even more so at their annual ball at the University in the spring term where they and their partners danced the lancers, reels and the highland schottische, attired as they were in full dress uniform with white spats, red flashes and their hose tops, Gordon tartan kilts, red tunics and large tartan plaids.*

Lawrence continued his studies at Aberdeen. By October 1914, *Alma Mater* was already commenting on the dwindling membership of the committees and clubs. In November 1914, Lawrence was elected president of the Students' Representative Council. In January 1915, he won the £5 James Anderson Gold Prize in Clinical Medicine.

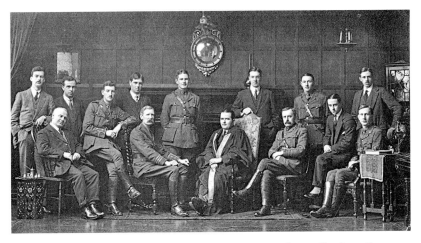

Lawrence as President of the Students' Representative Council, standing in uniform between the two men in the centre. Professor John Marnoch (in uniform) is seated left below Lawrence and Bernard Davies, President of the Union.

Early in 1915, when most of his friends were on active service, Lawrence completed his midwifery course. Thomas Lawrence had by this time inherited a share of uncle Brushy Morrison's wealth: 'he was always ready to spend money on the best education he could for me', and Lawrence was accepted as a student at the Coombe Lying-In Hospital, situated in the middle of the old slums of Dublin. After seeing two or three deliveries by expert midwives, and hearing a few excellent lectures on what to do, Lawrence was sent to help with a nearby delivery armed only with a pair of sterilized rubber gloves. He felt shaky with ignorance.

> However, as I climbed the stairs I felt less nervous and soon the baby was delivered, gave a tremendous yell, greeted the world, and no wonder: to be suddenly brought from a warm intra-uterine bath into the cold room where, whether from poverty or thoughtlessness, no clothing for the babe was available. The priests were very prompt to baptize an infant into the Holy Roman Church but did nothing I could see for its terrestrial welfare. When I went there the next morning to take the woman's temperature and to see the baby, I was told that after giving the child its first breast feed she went off to her work as usual, leaving the baby with friendly neighbours who did well until afternoon when, unnerved by the continuous yells of hunger, they persuaded her husband to bring her back early to resume her parental duties, hoping that he would do some work for a change to provide the necessary food and Guinness.
>
> The sterile rubber gloves, if one obeyed the instructions issued with them, prevented one's scratching first at the ankles, then the knees, then further up, caused by the ubiquitous attacks from wretched fleas. What a relief when every delivery was over to have a good scratch. The itching of flea bites continued all night and one got little sleep. Those Irish women were certainly tough.

Lawrence then always carried a roll of warm flannel for the babes, although he could ill afford it on his allowance. He notes that there was not a great deal on which to spend one's pocket money in Dublin in those days. He didn't like Guinness, and entertainments, such as 'the excellent theatre', were half-price for Coombe students.

Lawrence completed the necessary 20 domiciliary deliveries, but, before leaving, the Coombe students were invited to a sing-song by the mainly Irish students at the Rotunda, the other lying-in hospital. The Rotunda was in the middle of Dublin's West One, with no slums:

> And how their students could learn to practise the difficulty and variabilities of midwifery we could not grasp. However, our all-Irish hosts were very hospitable, and asked me, as a recognised pianist, to open the musical evening, which I did by playing as loudly and as accurately as I could on an out-of-tune piano. Loud cheers, but undeserved I felt. Then some lovely Irish lyrics, from deep Irish voices. The music I found easy to play. So the evening went on with intervals for drinks – not entirely Guinness, I am glad to say. When it was nearly midnight and thinking it was time to go, I played God Save the King which was lustily sung by the overseas students but there was not a murmur from the Irish, who were probably hearing it for the first time.

We went down the street in a pretty merry mood and in front of us was a splendid, highly coloured, advertising sign 'The Cosy Corner Cinema'. This was too inviting to be left untouched, and two of our tallest got it down easily. We marched about with it on our shoulders along the street and deposited it on the steps of the smartest hotel in Sackville Street – the Park Lane of Dublin – where the porters regarded us as dangerous hooligans and must have telephoned the police. A bevy of police arrived, bursting with laughter when they saw the 'Cosy Corner Cinema' sign, but stern enough to take us to the Police Station for our names and addresses. 'The Coombe', we said with one voice. The Superintendent telephoned the hospital to see if we were genuine: 'Yes, they are; and we want them back quickly to help three women in labour, so please tell them to hurry back, Inspector, sir.' But how could we, not knowing Dublin or where we were? But as we came in, I saw a swift Police car warming up for action. 'Do you think, sir, you could hurry us to the Coombe in five minutes and then hurry back to chase any real criminals you may want to catch? Then I shall go to Glasgow tomorrow with happy memories of an amusing and harmless last evening in Dublin and of the humanity of the Irish police.' He thought and nodded, blew a blast on his whistle which brought the car to the door for orders. 'Please, Murphy, take these doctors to the Coombe as quickly as you can and then come back here.' As we left, we waved vigorously and sang 'For he's a jolly good fellow.' Drive carefully was not in Murphy's vocabulary and I was thankful to arrive safely at The Coombe in less than five minutes.

He returned from Dublin to resume his medical studies and to keep in touch with his friends serving abroad.

In April 1915, Lawrence was recovering from another infection, and during this convalescence he was deeply saddened to hear that after only a few weeks in France, Charlie Macrae had been shot dead through the heart by a sniper outside his trench in France when he was bending down to give assistance to a comrade. The entry in the University Roll of Honour records that the sniper's bullet ended a career of unusual possibilities, for Charlie had a 'brain and a personality that might have carried him to the top of almost any ladder he chose to climb'. Two days later, another friend, Stuart Paterson, who was in the same battalion as Charlie, was also killed by a sniper. Both men were buried at Wytschaete Cemetery in Belgium. Lawrence kept their obituaries from the newspaper and their personal letters for the rest of his life.

On 18 May 1915, Lawrence's great friend and neighbour from Aberdeen,

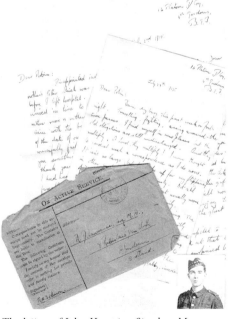

The letters of John Hampton Strachan Mason known as Jack.

Jack Mason, ex-Editor of the *Alma Mater*, wrote to him from Flanders. Jack had graduated with honours in English in 1911 before being involved in literary work in London in 1914. Lawrence was convalescing at home and in Ballater, but was experiencing war through Jack's letters, which would be quite unlike anything reported in the Aberdeen press. Jack appreciated Lawrence's interest in his wartime experiences, since most other friends avoided the topic. He was quite severe about Lawrence's recent letter:

> As the letter of a still sick man it really ought to have been more stimulating. I can perceive in it fleeting suggestions of morbidity powerfully suppressed. A paragraph beginning 'Our lives just now must be one of huge contrast' should have been a sheer delight. But it petered out before you had made even the vaguest attempt to define my life. Intuition be damned, sir, and pusillanimity also!

During this particular letter writing session, Jack came under direct fire but then picked up his pen again to tell Lawrence how the dug-out next to theirs was 'blown to blazes by a whiz bang'. He went on to say that just after that episode he developed a 'slight seediness', which in fact was to keep him out of action several weeks. He wrote again when he had just been discharged from a month in hospital and had missed being in the trenches at Ypres, or the 'Hell's Cauldron' as he called it, in which 'the battalion goose was being cooked' on the front line. He thought it was quite possible that he owed his life to that period in hospital, for the tales his comrades from the remnants of D Company told him made a profound impression. Jack, who, like many of the ex-university soldiers had chosen not to accept a commission, brought Lawrence up to date with news of their mutual acquaintances also told him that Lawrence's mother had taken the trouble to send

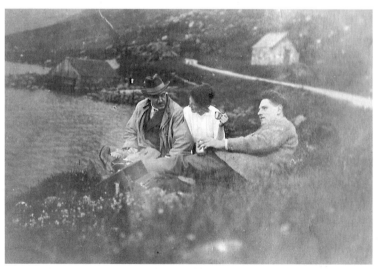

Lawrence's convalescence near Ballater, probably on the shores of Loch Muick in 1915: sipping tea from dainty china cups.

him a letter and 'edibles, drinkables and fumables': 'I am in hopes from what she said that you will now be recovering in something of a fit state to enjoy the sun and countryside. It's about time that ghost of your appendix had ceased to haunt you.'

In July 1915, Lawrence had written a piece called 'The Washing of the Waster' in the *Alma Mater* that seemed to have been an amusing account of his experiences in the nursing home and from which it seems he wondered if his decision to go into Surgery was wise. Jack wrote in reply:

> It is blithering funny to think of your reflections on the theme (of a Waster). The kinema makes great sport of the flabby, innocent sedentary old gentleman compelled by circumstances to a whirlwind of activity but there is a lot of comedy too in my picture of you, a young Apollo, snared – bound while war and the world wage on without you.
>
> … Go easy and if you have to chuck the thought of specialising in surgery so much the better. You have always 'Kingseat' [a mental hospital] to resort to. I shall always be able to follow your mental processes and results more easily there than in the operating theatre of the Infirmary.

Lawrence would learn more about life on the front near Ypres when Jack analysed fear in minute detail in response to Lawrence's probing questions on fear and fatalism. Jack was 23, a year older than Lawrence at the time of writing, yet the letters have the maturity and insight of a much older man:

> July 27th 1915 … Fear is the most degrading of the emotions. I know a lot about it now but have made no anatomy of it. It isn't what I thought it would be. Excitement, nervous tension, go by the name of 'fear' often, but that is merely 'fright' – a different matter altogether. I confused the two before and used to think myself a greater coward than now I know I am. Fear is the instinct that prompts the stretcher bearer to seek cover behind his loaded stretcher. Fear encourages you to find some excuse at all costs to remain in safety if the danger is without the trench or to escape from it if the danger is within. It is degrading to find yourself willing to sacrifice anybody for the sake of your life. Education which increases one's self-respect, increases on the average, one's stock of courage. Apart from the efficacy of pride to overcome fear, common sense often keeps it at arm's length. But pure fear is too primitive to allow of much being said. The curious results in the mind of the presence of physical danger are more interesting in subtler ways.
>
> Once a man has learnt himself he has learnt everything. From the point of view of the world it is more tragic that a man should die at 24 than that he should die at 70. From the point of view of the individual it is possibly preferable. What he might have taught others will largely perish with him but the most interesting part of his work is already done or half done … I am sorrier for the youngsters who die than for those nearer my own age. The years back and forward about twenty are so glorious. Once a man has begun to declare himself he has begun to die. My fatalism as you call it is either not very necessary to me or it is most thoroughly pervasive and deep seated. For the truth is, I never trouble very much about fate and the future. The

present which is 'I' contents and fills me and I do not value my life except for the living of it. To die is not a verb which has any bearing on life, that which is terrible in life is not to die but to succumb to fear.

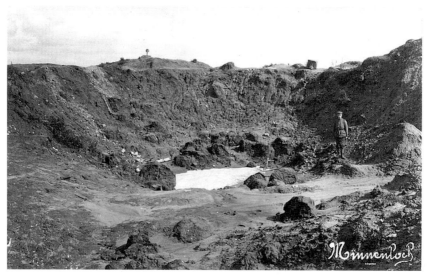

The crater at Hooge, photographed in 1915 by Dr Trenkler.

Mason explained to Lawrence how:

Rifle bullets are endurable without much shock to the nerves, they are invisible and the sound they make comparatively slight. Besides there is the feeling that they can only snaffle one man. A small shell is really less dangerous than mild rifle fire but is much more exciting and so by degrees of sound up to the explosion of an aerial torpedo which is a long cylinder that climbs quite visibly nodding slowly up in the air, curves steeply, and comes down like a rocket to explode like a mine. The noise of a big explosion I think in most cases has most to do with getting the wind up. After the explosion it is possible to localise it by sight but not by sound. Therefore I am always happier when I can see where shells are landing even when I cannot see but have to depend wholly on my ears although I may be reasonably certain that they are not very near.

He described the effect of being under shell fire to Lawrence:

The nervous loss can continue to prostration after this point. What one thinks about during those moments I do not know. It is quite inarticulate, a waiting ... It is possible to sit under an inferno of shells and be quite calm. I have never done so, but I know that I could do what every other man in the company did. And the last time I was in the trenches a British mine was exploded about two or three hundred yards away to be succeeded by attacks and counter attacks and artillery duel of a few hours. Our trench escaped the shelling by some inexplicable miracle but we were waiting for our turn all the time. Yet I was dancing with excitement and would willingly have charged the whole German army single-handed. The din was so terrific, the spectacle so huge that the limitations of my five foot six of human clay were utterly transcended, its violability forgotten and I became the creator and the destroyer, the evening and the earth.

He asks Lawrence if these musings were 'very original, very vapid or very different from what I might have said in the years "ante bellum"?' The letter ended by saying that he was not afraid of death but still afraid of dying. Having read so many detailed descriptions of life under fire, Lawrence might have been surprised to read Mason's conclusion:

My last reflection on me and the war. I never enjoyed any months of my life better than these in Flanders – not by a long way so well.

Mason was a member of a The Jocks' Society in the 4th Gordons. These intelligent young men were missing the stimulus of academic life. Many carried copies of Houseman's *A Shropshire Lad* in their battledress pocket. They organized meetings, and one member, Robert Stewart, wrote it was 'a genuine University gathering – for we were wont to assemble in rest billets, after our day's work was done, and forget Belgium and its mud, in sweet retrospection'. Stewart also recorded that at their last meeting, which was held on 22 September 1915 over a supper of potatoes and meat sauce:

The speeches of Privates Mason and Surtees were received with keen relish, and appreciated as delicacies by their hearers … Supper over, we gathered round the heart of the open fireplace and the past occupied our thoughts. Marischal College, with all its joys and associations, was discussed, and many a wish expressed that soon, notebook in hand, we would again cross the quadrangle. No mention of the morrow was made.

In his enforced state of idleness, Lawrence was able through these detailed and vivid accounts to experience their activities at second hand. He was all too aware that he could have been with those 4th Gordons in Flanders. These letters from Lawrence's friends were probably cathartic for the writers, who were able to say things to a friend of the same age that they would have shrunk from revealing to their parents. It was also a way of retaining some contact with normal life. We can only imagine Lawrence's bitter grief when he received news of Jack Mason's death at Hooge in the Battle of Loos on 25 September, three days after giving that speech to the Society. Walter Inkster, cartoonist and fellow tennis team member, also died on the 25th. The combined casualty list of the 1st and 4th Gordons on that shocking day was 32 officers and 635 other ranks killed and wounded. A colleague wrote that Mason's death came as a terrible shock: 'It seemed so short a time since he had been one of ourselves.'

They carry back bright to the coiner the mintage of man,
  The lads that will die in their glory and never be old.

From *A Shropshire Lad*

That September day was a dark one for Aberdeen; at least 15 ex-students were killed at Hooge – 'a type of collective experience not undergone by universities with OTCs whose members were dispersed'. Of the 120 rank-and-file soldiers who went from Bedford to Flanders, there were only three left in the ranks. Later in 1917, when he was Rector of Aberdeen University, Winston Churchill wrote:[5]

The extraordinary reputation acquired by the Scottish divisions in our army which was already represented as the flower of our race in all parts of the world was due in no small degree to the astonishing military and personalities of the young Scottish gentlemen who hastened from the Universities to command and lead their countrymen in the field. Aberdeen University will rightly cherish their memory and its most precious possession.

Lawrence was never able to talk about his friends from the ill-fated Gordon Highlanders without tears in his eyes. He kept a photograph of them on his desk until the end of his life and the letters from Jack Mason and his other friends were kept carefully preserved among his personal possessions.

Lawrence continued to be *hors de combat* because of the recurring infections, which required surgery. On 11 July 1915, Robert Forgan wrote from the trenches in northern France, where he was serving in the RAMC:

I am damnably sorry for you, Robbie Doo. That you may soon be well on the high road to health and that this 3rd op. may really be a means of accelerating your ultimate complete recovery is, I am sure, the wish of very many people, and not least of, Ponto.

He later wrote about a close shave:

22nd July 1915 ... I was dashed near it though, a few weeks ago, for a shell dropped about 20 yards away from

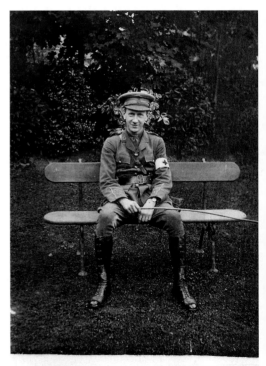

Robert Forgan (Ponto).

where I was tending a wounded man who'd been struck by a shell 5 minutes before. It's a queer sensation – a terrific bang, a cloud of black smoke and flying bits of shell and road. Two stones hit me and I wondered if I were wounded, but my tunic wasn't even torn. I got a hell of a fright but the necessity of looking after the wounded man gave my rattled nerves a chance of recovery.

Lawrence (now a Lieutenant) remained in Aberdeen during October 1915 and achieved success during the academic year 1915–16 by winning the Shepherd Memorial Gold Medal in Surgery. In October 1915, he was back in hospital for surgery under Professor Marnoch. Forgan wrote, 'Today I have got news of you which makes me very disappointed with you. In spite of all my exhortations you have not got completely cured and so, poor lad, you appear to have been once more subjected to the tender mercies of Johnny and Co.' In later life, Lawrence wondered whether the repeated episodes of peritonitis and low-grade sepsis caused a cyst in the pancreas and subsequent diabetes. He wanted, but did not get, a post-mortem to satisfy his scientific theory posthumously.

The *Alma Mater* had become a much slimmer publication by 1915. It was now run almost exclusively by women and was only being produced monthly instead of weekly. An editorial in the December issue noted, 'Our best have gone from us, our classrooms are half empty', but went on to urge students to keep the societies going. A letter from Lawrence was published in the November 1915 edition:

Dear Sir
This hardly seems a time for suggesting innovations, however slight in the Medical curriculum, but is a better thing for seed to fall on barren ground than not to fall at all, and really, as this war has nothing to do with it, the soil is as fertile as it ever will be.

Everybody will admit that a doctor must earn a living, and it is a sad fact that he leaves the University knowing nothing about financial aspects of his profession and various subjects of social importance. He has no idea what to charge his patients; how to keep books or have them kept. More important, he knows nothing about panel matters and has but a vague idea of medical etiquette. He is thus sure to make unnecessary preliminary blunders.

Now Professor Hay, our University financier has recently dropped from his Course on Medical Jurisprudence some dozen lectures on public health. As 'death from drowning' does not seem to be very popular just now, and crime, in Britain at least, is in decline, there seems no need to lengthen the descriptions of such matters. Three or four lectures on the above subjects would be all that would be necessary, and here we have the time, the place and the Professor all together.

So if fellow Medical Students see eye to eye in this matter, let us be up and doing. A word in the right place should be enough.

I am sir, yours etc. RD Lawrence

A few weeks later, he spoke in the debate, 'Are our Scottish Universities fulfilling their proper function?'

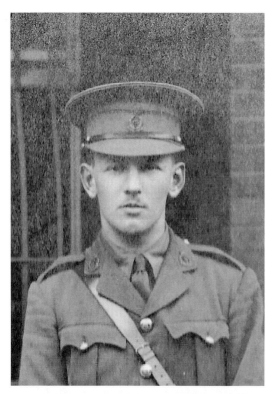
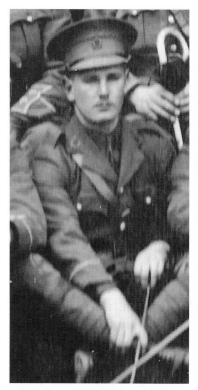
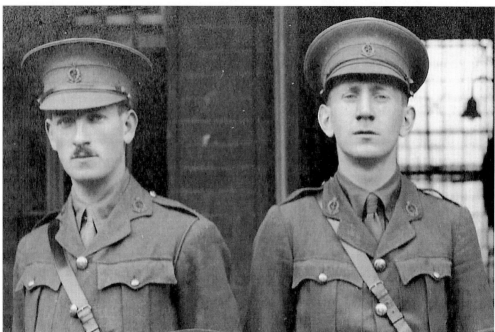

Aldershot 1914 – RAMC Officers (clockwise from top left) Tom Menzies, RD Lawrence, Robert Forgan and Robert B Myles.

Meanwhile on the Western Front, Arthur Landsborough Thomson, who was attached to the 11th Argyll and Sutherland Highlanders in France, wrote to Lieutenant R. D. Lawrence at home in Aberdeen in October 1915, giving him another idea of what life under fire in the trenches was like:

I was most sorry to hear you had had another relapse and operation and missed your Final again. A more cheering piece of news was that you were standing it all as well as ever and that something probably radical had been found and righted this time. I must fervently hope this is true. I have asked my people to let me have any news of you they hear. But perhaps you'll write yourself before long.

I have been with this Kitchener battalion for a month now and any antagonism they had to an intruder from an SR unit has long ago worn off. They are a very good crowd really and the Division did great things in the big advance. We are going into the trenches for twelve days tomorrow after a week's comparative ease and comfort. Our last spell of a week was pretty 'hot'. For the three days we had in the front line we scarcely ate or slept and were heavily bombarded with every manner of projectile from the bullet to the aerial torpedo and from hand bomb to Jack Johnsons [a large artillery shell]. I was very lucky to go unscathed when our trench (a rotten ditch of a thing won a few days before) was flattened out by high explosive quite near me and a lot of my platoon buried (extricated – not much the worse in most cases, however).

In the support trenches we had dug outs to sleep in and a pretty quiet time except when out in the open at night digging … I met several people I knew at the Base but only one at the front. By an extraordinary coincidence this one was Ponto (Robert Forgan)! He was shifted 15 miles south a month ago and now is just on our left. It is difficult to keep in touch but I unearthed him for the second time yesterday and expect him for dinner tonight. Get well quick! Write when you can, Yours ever LandsB

Forgan suggested an idea for the friends to keep in touch but sought Lawrence's approval for it first. He wrote:

'I like letter writing – it is an antidote to loneliness and serves to keep up friendships which might otherwise lapse. By the way, I want in some way to keep in touch with the four or five lads with whom I was more intimate. It is a sentimental notion – this of mine – but if every three months or six months each of us wrote a letter giving an account of what he'd been doing for the information and amusement of the other and sent it to some one of us who would act as secretary or editor or whatever you like to call it, we could have a very interesting document circulated every 3 or 6 months which would do something to keep us together.

I'm quite willing myself to undertake any secretarial work connected with such a scheme. And if you think it is practicable and give it your approval I shall explain the idea to the other lads. I suggest Bud, Boulton, LandsB, Bert,[6] yourself and me.

Forgan's idea was a stroke of genius and it took off. None knew what the future might bring – they had already lost many of their friends – but giving a date three months hence when the next summary was required must have given them a sense of purpose and a view of the future. Over the next two years, the group sent Forgan their news and he laboriously copied it out using carbon paper on thin, shiny army-issue paper and then circulated it to the group. This was tweeting 1915-style, and he called himself 'The Office Boy', directing what came to be known as 'Ponto's Bible Group'. The letters contain vivid accounts of life in many theatres of the war – France, the Mediterranean, Dardanelles and India – and have a strong streak of gallows humour running through them. From Aberdeen, Lawrence could experience vicariously the experiences of his friends. His contribution has not survived, but the set of letters remained folded in the family archive for 90 years.

Bud (McNeil) related:

I have now bathed in Alexandria, Malta, Mudros and off Anzac (Gallipoli Peninsula) and the only really good place is off Anzac. It's simply great after sweltering down in the wards amongst the stink of gas gangrene and dysentery to slip in off the gangway into the most perfect blue God ever made.

On leave in Aberdeen, McNeil wrote:

Landsbuggar's off to France … Robin when last I saw him was recovering or at least starting to recover from what I heard Johnnie thought was to be his last operation. He is as fat as any jug I ever saw and looking remarkably healthy.

Forgan himself described life in Northern France, where he had lodged briefly with a farming family whose baby had a large boil. He wrote:

A supper of omelette, bread and wine, the omelette consisting of 13 eggs owing to the good wife's misunderstanding the French of the man who ordered it – the said goodwife's baby's bottom, which had an enormous boil on it, successfully operated on by myself – and a 'cabinet' whose ammoniacal aroma haunts me still, and whose 30 foot shaft leading to the farmyard midden (which drained into the farmyard well) at the time struck me as a suitable rendezvous for mothers with infanticidal tendencies. French farmhouses must be seen (and smelt) to be believed.

LandsB in France summed up the curious mixture of emotions brought on by wartime experiences:

So I am at least standing it well. But I don't enjoy it, not one in ten thousand does. I wouldn't have missed it for worlds but it can stop as soon as it likes now I've seen it! There's damned little fun for an infantryman, during the winter anyway.

Boulton-Myles serving in India participated in the letterwriting scheme with some diffidence:

I beg to point out that it's a cold, hard, haemorrhoidally disposing world! Here am I on the 10th May faced with a terse and pointed notification from our prize maker of history and breaker of all rules and most hearts, that I have precisely 15 days in which to make up, think out, write down, read through, finish off, send on and cause to be delivered up in Aberdeen, a lengthy epistle of startling adventures replete with literary gems commensurate with a burnished intellect, wherewith to lighten the heavy hours and strew with roses the thorny couches of my trench ridden comrades …

In a personal letter to Lawrence, he also recorded a sentiment that was probably shared by many young RAMC doctors. He said that for most of his time serving in recent weeks in India, 'It was difficult to make out what the blighters were suffering from.'

From Forgan, we hear about Lawrence's graduation:

I refer to Robin's brilliant exit from the Varsity, trailing with him clouds of glory (or at least several stars.) But in spite of all his stars the way he behaved subsequently can hardly be called 'the milky way'. The revels commenced immediately on the declaration of the results and it was a great sight to see Lawrence proceeding up Union Street in a taxi kissing his hand to every girl he passed. Later on the Athenaeum and His Majesty's Theatre were the scenes of very audible jollifications.

I next met Rob at Heddington – the lad coming down for a night from Edinburgh. He was the sole guest of the Mess – it was Guest Night and with a fat cigar or a large thirst he mightily impressed the subalterns who wondered who the distinguished looking stranger might be.

The last letter that survives from the group was from June 1916 by LandsB, who wrote:

I rejoined my battalion when they were in the trenches of a certain notorious redoubt which we knew in quieter days before Xmas. On reaching the transport lines I heard that the Staff Captain was unable to get away to finish his interrupted leave as expected and that I had to return to my ordinary duties. And here was I decked out in new riding breeches and very new field boots and spurs. To preserve my dignity I said that I intended to ride up to the trenches: a desperate measure! That may not strike you as being very daring. But, think you, I was not born on a farm but in a city slum. Nor have I attended riding schools at Aldershot. Indeed I had never been on a horse in my life! However I sensed an animal whose spirit was long since broken and was content to carry me along at a dignified walk for which the cobbled road afforded an excuse. The Transport Officer, however, came along, and flicked the brute into sudden energy causing me to flatten my testicules [sic] into the semblance of identity discs. But I was so busy talking to the Transport Officer that I forgot to fall off. The episode gave me confidence although I felt the need of a suspensory bandage for the rest of the way. But it was quite a relief when the three miles were at an end and we were safely under fire once more instead of risking our lives on horseback.

Forgan and I haven't ceased to marvel at the luck which has thrown us in Divisions which are side by side since his move fifteen miles south seven weeks ago. Not counting the Base, he is the only man I've met here that I knew before, even slightly. We've had four meetings already. Yesterday I dined in his Chateau and tomorrow he dines in my cottage. After he goes on leave these meetings may cease.

Lawrence had finally graduated on 28th March 1916 with Second-Class honours, and Tom Menzies congratulated him on the 'splendid finish he has made by getting 2 stars in spite of his lengthy enforced idleness and subsequent amorous episodes with ladies of the boards and boarding houses.'

By October 1916, Lawrence was fully recovered and ready for what would be a very different war experience from that of his friends.

References

1. Quoted by Aristotle. *Rhetoric*, 1.7.34, 1365a.
2. The Fife Jameson medal was awarded to a student 'who shall distinguish himself most highly in a special competitive examination'.
3. *Oxford Dictionary of National Biography* entry, by David Evans.
4. McConachie J. *The Student Soldiers*. Elgin: Moravian Press, 1995.
5. A total of 2852 Aberdeen University staff, students and alumni served in the First World War, of whom 341 lost their lives. Their service spanned all branches of the Armed Forces. Many enlisted in the University's U Company of the 4th Gordons, others served with the Argyll and Sutherland, Seaforth, and Cameron Highlanders, as well as other army regiments and corps, the Royal Navy, Royal Army Medical Service, and the fledgling Royal Flying Corps. They came from all walks of life, all professions and ages – the youngest to die was only 18, the oldest was 66. Some died in the first weeks of the war, while others, haunted by battlefield illness and the horrors of the Front, lived on for some months after the armistice only to die after returning home. (Details are from *In Memoriam*, the Aberdeen University Roll of Honour.)
6. Herbert Sorley (1892–1968): he was at Aldershot with Lawrence and Boulton-Myles, and later became a colonial administrator.

CHAPTER 4

All Quiet on the North West Frontier

I wish I was going up Deeside instead of the Khyber.

RDL, 1919

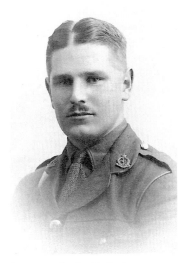

I n October 1916, the newly qualified 23-year-old Lawrence, recently restored to health after his illnesses, set sail on the troopship *Miltiades*[1] en route for Mesopotamia. Although straight out of medical school, he was the Senior Medical Officer (SMO) on board and therefore responsible for the health of a large number of troops. Lawrence's parents now had both sons serving in the RAMC. It must have put them in a state of anguish seeing their adored younger son set sail. There had been a slow drawing down of blinds all across Aberdeen and they would have known many of the 22 young men in their sons' close circle who had been killed.

Lawrence, Senior Medical Officer, 1916.

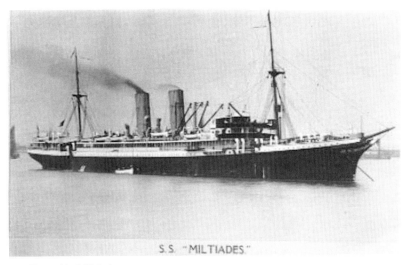

S.S. "MILTIADES"

HM Troopship Miltiades.

The younger son reassured his mother that the ship was 'going a very long way round to avoid submarines'. It was to travel via Cape Town, as the Mediterranean and Suez Canal were too heavily patrolled with German submarines. In the early part of the voyage, no lights were permitted on the ship after dark. He wrote with pride that despite tossing, pitching, rolling and wallowing on the briny waves and being surrounded by seasick troops and officers, he never missed a single meal or skipped any of his duties. He also noted how much sleep he had had since his illness – mostly 10 hours every night – and was never disturbed by the ship's heaving motion. He put his resistance to seasickness down to having a 'very stable nervous system'. He wrote that it had been great fun watching the fate of various officers at mealtimes, the looks of uncertainty, the whiteness and cold sweats, and the sudden disappearances.

He told his mother that his most interesting case was 'a morphinomaniac who has been taking enough morphia every day to kill ten ordinary men, but he'll have to give it up here, because neither he nor we have got enough stuff to keep him going even though we wished to'. Lawrence reassured his family that he had fallen on his feet again in quarters, in food, in health and ability to resist Neptune, and in being a SMO, and that he had just become a Captain. A week later, he wrote again:

to continue the fairy tale and it looks more like a fairy tale now, for we are now in the sub tropics and nearing the Tropic of Cancer and all those names which schooldays implanted in my memory, but which are now being revived and impressed upon me for the first time. I can't say where we are but it must be pretty evident by this time. The boat is settling down and the yellow seasick faces are creeping back to meals and sun and rosiness.

Life on board was entirely pleasurable:

One of the drafts aboard has discovered an orchestra which kept us bright and entertained at dinner and afterwards, though I think it is hardly fair to impose the well known waltzes of many a dance and

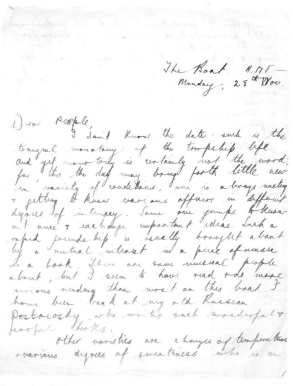

Example of a letter from Lawrence. He took pride in his handwriting and would later rue the fact that this wasn't a common feature with doctors.

Cinderella upon us lonely bachelors. … So life is bright and fair as it can be and I do not feel the monotony which many complain of, occupying my time quite satisfactorily with a little work, some reading of Thackeray and a desultory novel and much lying on my back in the sea breezes. The men are bucking up a bit now and beginning to sing, which is always a sign of the barometer.

He wrote again on 16 November:

We are creeping further and further south and have been through many variations in temperature since I last wrote. One morning we plunged into broiling sun with not a cloud in the sky and not a tiny breeze to take the sweat away. We all sweated pretty freely and drank iced drinks and ate less and lay about and did as little as possible. I began to get accustomed to it by the third day and grew less lazy but it does make me very lifeless.

We have had a busy time inoculating and have about finished 4000 now, so we shall have more time to ourselves now.

He was in charge of 80 men from the RAMC and gave them lectures on tropical diseases:

so that they will know something about them when they arrive. Sometimes I play the piano and sometimes I read and talk and sleep a very great deal. I eat hugely and am getting fat, so that I shall have a large store to draw on in case of necessity.

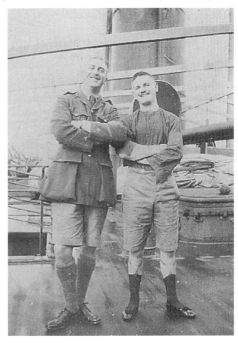

After three weeks, the ship arrived at Cape Town, which Lawrence described as

the most picturesque town I have ever seen. The wonderful Table Mountain dominating everything, the bright blue sea with the town neatly nestling between the two, white and clean with handsome buildings and gardens full of gorgeous flowers, some well known home favourites but huge and exotic in their growth, others quite new and semi-tropical, I suppose.

In Durban, Lawrence transhipped to the Castle Line *Kinfaun's Castle*,[2] 'a better boat than last. We are going to Bombay via German East Africa so I shall be far travelled soon. We leave troops at GEA (German East Africa) and go on. Some of the officers are waiting here for the next boat and they will have a lovely time, bathing and all sorts of profuse

Colleagues Doc and Stein with the shiny party pumps on board HMT Miltiades.

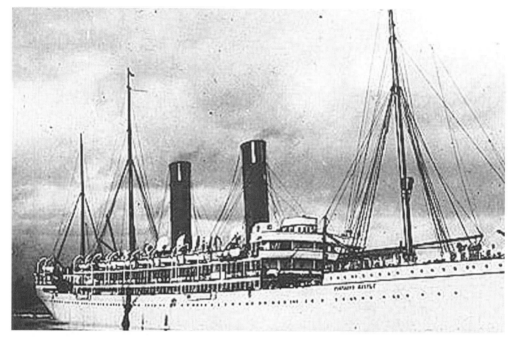

RMS Kinfaun's Castle.

hospitality.' He was in the dark about his eventual destination, but thought it was likely to be Mesopotamia, which largely corresponds to modern Iraq.

In fact, Lawrence had a lovely time on *Kinfaun's Castle*, writing that

I have long siestas in the afternoon and really the work is not trying. The food is very good and varied here and we are now having some fine South African fish and fruit which is a welcome change. We get an occasional wireless message to inform us of the condition of the war, but most people take more interest in talk and food and drinks than anything else. This is a very fine boat and rides along much faster than the old Miltiades. She is far more spacious and comfortable in most respects and holds another thousand troops. We have had some extraordinarily fine sunsets lately and they tell me the sunrises are finer still.

The only irritation was that he had to censor the troop's letters:

At first it rather interested me to read their letters and see them bragging or whining or making the best of it as the case may be, but the novelty soon passes off and most of the letters are the same.

On 7 December he wrote:

Just a further line to let you know that we are approaching our destination and shall there learn what is going to happen to us. It is an open question whether we stay

a short time in Bombay or go on straight to Mesopotamia. I should like to have a look round Bombay with David Walker, (an Aberdeen friend who was editor of the Times of India *in Bombay), and the probability is that we shall have at least one or two days even if this ship is going straight on there, as I suppose it needs coal and food. About the latter question, there is going to be a scandal and we have had a Board of Enquiry which has shown beyond doubt that the ship has been making money off the men's food. I hope those responsible get it thick and strong.*

He appreciated how lucky he was with this distant posting, when those of his contemporaries who had not already been killed were embroiled in the slaughter of the Battle of the Somme while his own life glided on pleasantly. He seemed unaware of the extremely difficult conditions for the British Army in Mesopotamia. He regarded it as an opportunity for some sport:

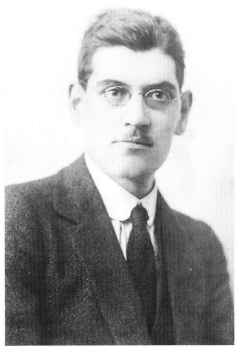

David Walker (1892–1926). [Editor Times of India. *Won the Amateur Golf Championship of India.]*

This is a splendid time to be going to Mespot. I am going to buy a sporting gun as there is abundant duck shooting they tell me and also a store of fishing tackle to lure the wily fish, as much with a view to a change of food as amusement and sport. I shall also take some quick growing vegetables and see what can be done in the way of market gardening.

However, things were very different from this:[3]

A more difficult theatre in which to fight would be hard to imagine. Flies and mosquitoes attacked the troops, many of whom became sick. Soldiers froze during the winter nights, and were overcome by heat during the summer. Dust turned to mud when the banks of the Tigris overflowed during the rainy season.

The ship arrived in Bombay in December 1916 and, in Lawrence's own words, he fell on his feet. When he went to the Disembarkation Medical Officer, he found 'a bosom friend', Bud Rose from Aberdeen, acting in that capacity during the absence of his chief. Rose asked where he was going, to which Lawrence replied that he thought it would be Mesopotamia. Rose could not find any orders and 'on talking over the matter he thought I had better not go to Mespot even though the climate and place is quite agreeable at this time of year. So he wired the Director

Medicinal Service of India how to dispose of me and he seems to think I shall be posted somewhere in India.'

Rose offered to put Lawrence up in his flat, but the afternoon was free and he got his first impression of India:

I got into a gharry [horse drawn vehicle] with another officer and went to a bank to change money. It was an open Victorian affair and we had good fun getting the driver to go where we wanted or thought we wanted. It was pretty hot but not very oppressively so, and our eyes were kept hard at work on all the strange sights on the streets. Natives in thousands; brown men with white clothes swathing their legs, bright coloured band round their waists; some in European white trousers; most with bare feet, some with sandals, or shoes, and some even rising to socks; some with waist clothes alone; some with red or black fezzes or white turbans or practically bare shaven heads; lots of children quite naked and Parsee women in the most gorgeous shades of orange and scarlet or purple and white with long veils. They have a fine erect carriage and a swinging gait and many of the poorer women had copper vessels on their head or a bundle of clothes. Everything weird and fantastic, nothing known or expected from our point of view. And the buildings were all very white and everything bright and dazzling, while, the most striking of all, in every corner, on the pavements, in gutters, at shop doors, sat hundreds of natives doing nothing but gazing calmly on the busy street. They tell me that they are Micawbers waiting for some job to turn up.

By 10 December he knew that he would be staying in India and going to the Peshawar Division 'but there is no word yet which station'. He was delighted with the posting and felt it was 'about the best place I could be going to: cold and bracing at this time of year and a most interesting place'. He assured his mother that there was no active service there, and asked her to send him 'all kinds of clothes', enclosing a list of outfits more suited to a spell of imperial peacetime duties: 'mess kit, complete. White shirts, collars etc., khaki trousers and breeches, field boots, tennis things, dressing gown, silver cigarette case, grey lounge suit, shirts – all decent ones I have, golf suit and stockings and fawn cap, dinner jacket and studs and music songs.' As an afterthought, he added, 'Also Hewlitt's *Bacteriology* from the study. I shall probably be here some days yet and then I travel the length of India before I get to my destination. Thus life is very rosy.'

In this rosy life, he had fallen among his old Aberdeen friends. Lawrence and Walker with their friend Rose went in a gharry the 2½ miles to Rose's digs, which were on the promenade overlooking the sea. New to India, Lawrence was overwhelmed by the colours:

The sea is calm and beautiful, there is always a breeze except in the early morning, the sunsets are wonderful over the Governor's House, the moon is full just now making the sky and sea a heliotrope green at night and everywhere the colours are beyond your imagination because you haven't seen them. Perhaps you remember in Bowman's window in Union Street water colours of the pyramids and the desert? These colourings are very like it.

He continued with a description of their outing:

We went in Robertson's motor about 9.45 to the Taj Mahal, the famous hotel, to attend the weekly dance of the youth and beauty of Bombay. The night was luscious and we went in the motor without coat or hat clad in the lightest drill, mess kit and dinner jacket, according to our different station and wardrobe. It was a very gay sight, great mixture of people and good dancing. Bud Rose is quite in the swim and passed me on to some ladies who danced me round and I sweated and sweated and was very cheered after my long spell on the boat. Dining in state in the room overlooking the dancing was the Nazim of Hyderabad, the greatest Indian prince. They sat long watching the dancing more than anything else. About 11.20 we went to the Yacht Club, the finest in Bombay, overlooking the harbour and had some sandwiches in the loveliness of the moonlit night and the sparkling sea before going home about I a.m. very sleepy, but not too tired.

He then embarked on a journey to some of the most famous sights in India. With a servant 'a Mohammedan, one Sulim Sassani by name who has had much service with military men judging from the references he brought', he travelled from Bombay to Agra in 'a large broad gauge carriage more like the cabin of a ship than anything else, broad, airy, no corridor and long sleeping berths ... My servant travels just beside me.'

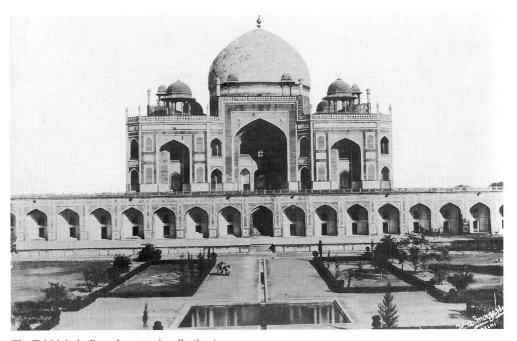

The Taj Mahal. (From Lawrence's collection.)

In Agra, he drove to the Taj Mahal at 11.30 pm and

was spell bound till 1.30 then home. It is the most mysterious beautiful stately, sedate and lovely thing ever I have known in man's handiwork. It seems quite unreal in its pale white beauty in the moonlight. Today I shall see it in detail at evening and also Agra fort and then go on to Delhi.

From Delhi, he went to Amritsar and

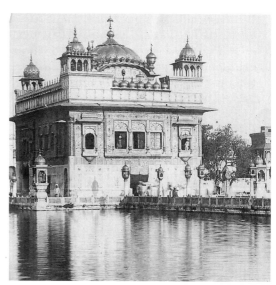

The Golden Temple at Amritsar.

slept all night as the carriage was just like beds when my boy has built them up. It would have been very cold without my flea bag and one blanket. As it was rosy slumber clothed my whole journey. I managed to get breakfast at the train before reaching Amritsar so that I wasted no time when I got there. I leapt into a 'tonga' which is a jolting flimsy kind of buggy very prevalent in this part of the world – and dashed off to see the sight of the place. That is the Golden Temple of the Sikhs, the holiest place in Amritsar, which is the chief centre of their religion. The Sikhs are the Puritans of the Hindus. They do not shave, nor smoke, nor cut their hair at all and these little eccentricities were the cause of much bloodshed and gory diversions between them and their neighbours before the British protected their religion. [At the temple] I had to take off my shoes and put on large flimsy boats of canvas, had to leave all my smoking impedimenta behind and I was somewhat surprised that I was not detained till my face and head

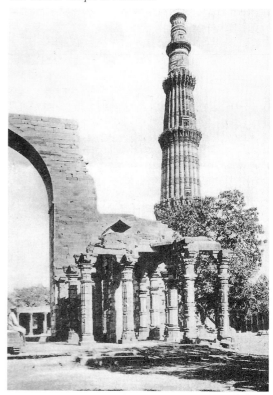

The Qutub Minar, Delhi, showing inscriptions and honeycombs.

had grown sufficiently hairy to appease the deity or that I had not to suffer the indignity of a wig.

I now got a Sikh policeman to take me round and I skirted the pool beside which numerous people were washing and bathing and got into the holy of holies where I was immediately made welcome by some Johnny throwing a garland round my neck. Everywhere there were flowers scattered in profusion and the whole aspect of the worship was simple and attractive. It went on in a marble hall about the size of our drawing room, but more open with arcade in the middle of the sides so that people could pass freely out and in. There seemed to be a sort of Bible from which someone read, but in his clothes he was indistinguishable from anyone else. The chair tickled and pleased me greatly and really was rather fine and impressive. Three bearded men, two with banjo-like instruments which they sawed like a fiddle and another fine looking blind fanatic banged away at tom toms usually very tunefully and quite subdued. Then one would break into a chanting kind of song in which I really could detect music in a minor key and which reminded me of some of the Tartar songs that used to accompany the Russian ballet dancers. Women in gorgeous colours of poor attire would come in, salaam proudly and scuttle off with a bit of a flower. No collection was required but there was a cloth on to which people threw small coins mostly the equivalent of 12th of a penny but I did the lordly Sahib with a rupee as no doubt was expected and only natural and in due proportion. The whole place is very gaudy with gold and cheap precious stones. I rather liked it.

He took the train for the short journey to Lahore and

came straight to the best hotel – I have always stayed in the best hotels all this trip. They said they had no room, so I got them to fit me up a tent in which I anticipate sleeping under about 50 blankets tonight. This afternoon I set out to do the sights of Lahore in a galloping tonga. The horses look desperately done up – you would choose out of the rustiest old cab horse at home as a galloper of far superior merit – but appearances are deception. My horse looked all bone, but must have been all sinew and heart, for he cantered and galloped up hills all the six miles to Shalamar. Does the name suggest anything to you? The song, 'Pale hands pink tipped'[4] brings in the word it certainly has got the atmosphere of the place also. It is a lovely garden inside high brick walls with fountains and lakes imprisoned in white marble and strewn with creamy minarets and tiny palaces.

His next letter was from the RAMC Mess Rawalpindi on 22 December:

Yesterday I travelled up through the Punjab from Lahore to Pindi through very wonderful country – flat dusty plains with the snow clad ranges of Himalayas about 100 miles away. The scenery is extraordinarily fine but very barren and inhuman, so different from homely little Scotland. Myles (Robert Boulton Myles – friend from University) met me at the station, just home from 3 weeks manoeuvres and looking very fit and not at all changed that I could see. He took me straight to his bungalow and then to the club and afterwards to mess – it being guest night. …

I have had a great tour through India and have seen most of the sights which are commonly prescribed for tourists.

He spent Christmas with his old friend Myles 'in a most cheery way'. He had been due to report at Peshawar on Sunday 24th, but took the executive decision not to spend Christmas (his first away from home) among complete strangers:

I thought no one would want me or expect me to turn up at that season – and I was right. So I passed the time in tennis, riding, golf, lunches and dinners and a dance and everything was bright and cheery as Myles introduced me to all I need know. Xmas day itself I spent in lunching with the Colonel, singing at a soldiers' home and Xmas dinner in the Mess where the officer's wives were being entertained. Thus two plum puddings were the results and I had little appetite next day. Did you all dine en famille *I wonder?*

After two months travel, he arrived in Peshawar at the end of December 1916. His first days there were very quiet so that

I hardly know what to do with myself all day yet. I wanted some tennis this afternoon but so far I have not been able to fix up any. So I shall look at the Urdu language for a short time, then visit my tailor – one Shah by name and then go to a cricket match. Sport seems to occupy the great part of one's life here, all the usual games and hunting and polo besides.

He ended on the reassuring note that 'this place is a health resort at this time of year'.

He wrote again on New Year's Eve to report:

I really started work this morning but there was not much to do and now I have the rest of the day to myself. I don't know what I shall do yet. Probably I'll go to the city in the after noon have a look at it. We English all live in the Cantonment about a mile away from the city and so far I have not seen anything of it. It is quite unsafe at night for a white man.

He went on to say:

I shall have to call on all sorts of people as it seems to be the custom to 'call' on practically everyone in the Cantonment. A call consists in going to a house and dropping cards in the box if you are lucky enough to find them out. I shall probably do some of that this afternoon.

Lawrence was meticulous about his weekly letter home. He particularly liked it when his mother asked him questions so that he could react to those rather than compose new, fresh reports of his routine and activities.

He described his bungalow in great detail and listed the large number of servants he had. Apart from the work with his patients, everything was done for him. The

British Empire was at its zenith and, as he commented in one letter, 'considering we are at the very boundary of civilization it is wonderful how like the life is to that in England'. A punkah-wallah kept him cool in his bedroom on hot summer nights. He had a servant to himself for 30 rupees a month (1 rup = 2 pence), and for this he was woken and served with tea in the morning. The servant cleaned everything, helped him dress, put his boots on, fastened his braces, kept the room clean, prepared his warm bath and waited upon him at meals. He did also note that they were all apt to be lazy and took a lot of looking after to keep up to scratch. They had always to salaam when they came into Lawrence's presence – all natives had to take off their shoes when they came into a white man's house as servants or tradesmen. With the team of 20 servants looking after him, we hear in a later letter how he evolved canny ways of managing them, very much in the imperial style:

Our gardener – indeed we have two, the gardener and his son – is a most lazy fellow and has to be hounded at the point of the boot. This is quite literal; otherwise he will do no work. The garden would grow any amount of vegetables, only the gardener (mali) doesn't think fit to do so. I invented rather a good plan for making him work. Any vegetable, which is in season and obtainable in the bazaar and yet is not in the garden, I buy from the bazaar and debit it to the mali's wages. He doesn't like this at all and since then there has been a marked improvement in quality and quantity of his produce. These arbitrary methods are the only ones which succeed here.

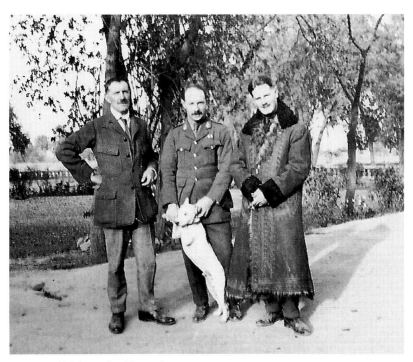

Lawrence (right) wearing his postin.

He went on to describe a typical day:

It is evening after mess and I am in my room in my bungalow before a fire of wood, wearing a large fur-coat, called a 'postin', These are yellow goatskin or sheepskin coats with the fur turned inside and the skin cured yellow and embroidered and trimmed with astrakhan. They are very large and warm and useful to slip off and on at night going to the mess from the bungalow and back. The system of living is the following. We eat in the mess and sit there in the day and it is a largish bungalow with a sitting room and a dining-room. It has quite a decent piano and is where we live. We all live in bungalows round about, each having a room and a bathroom attached. Now that we are at home you might send me your photos, please, to adorn the walls. The room is large and very high for the hot weather. It has two or three doors and windows and is rather cold this weather. However, I find five blankets keeps the cold out all night. I have got a British warm made lined with bearskin and several clothes which the native tailors make rather cheaply. I am going to buy some Indian goods to furnish my house when I come home, rugs and ornaments, perhaps some brass work and any curios I fancy very much. At any rate be sure that my room is quite comfortable now and a cheerful fire of wood of some sort is burning at my feet. I have plenty of time to myself and when I get properly settled down I mean to use it in doing some reading.

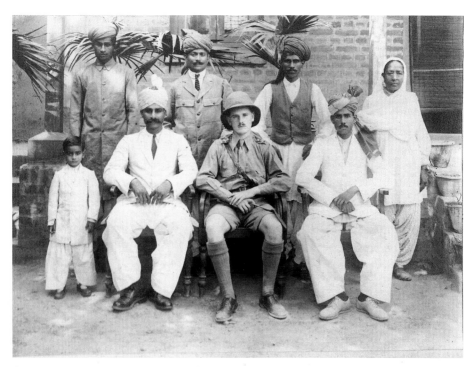

Nowshera Cantonment Hospital, 1917. Back (L to R): Abdul Ghami B., Misar Ali, Faqir Mohd., Umdan Matron. Front (L to R): S. Ahjaz Hussain, S. Walsyat Shah SAS, Capt. R. D. Lawrence RAMC, Lorinda Mall. (Annotated photograph from Lawrence's collection.)

The following will give you a rough idea of my day. I get up at 7.45, shave and dress rapidly in the bitter cold and walk about 10 minutes off in the Cantonment [military station, permanent camp] to the 2 Devon's Regiment whose MO I am. I do their sick parade at 8.30 and have a good many men. But before this I have a short walk to see the hills round the Khyber from a viewpoint very clear in the morning, frost with the snowy higher mountains behind them. After sick parade I usually come back for some breakfast and then go to my malaria ward in the hospital and see that all is right. After which I go to any officers of the Devons who may be sick in their quarters and fill in the rest of the morning reading or dropping cards on people. Lunch at one and then we are practically free for the day unless one is orderly officer and has to make a round of the hospital again or do any emergency job that may turn up. In the afternoon I sometimes play tennis and today I borrowed a pony and had a splendid canter on the race course. Most of the officers keep ponies here, but I don't think I shall do so on account of my tummy,[5] but will content myself with borrowing one occasionally. One has tea about five and lounges about, perhaps reads or talks and today I had my first [Urdu] lesson with a native teacher, one Mahometkhan by name. Mess is at 8.15 and the meal lasts about an hour and then music making slightly, or reading or chatting either in the mess or in the bungalow sees us in bed by twelve.

He wrote in January 1917 that he is

being shifted again and before I go I'll just drop a note to inform you of the fact. I'm going further away still to the D(urham) L(ight) (I)nfantry 1st Battalion. They are posted at an outpost fort Shabkadar about 17 miles north east of Peshawar right on the frontier. We sit behind barbed wire looking formidable and doing nothing, just waiting to see if a race of Pathans[6] called the Mohmands will come down and fire a few shots and then go back again.

Winston Churchill had served in the area and described the Pathans as 'Stone Age savages whose daily deeds are treachery and violence'. Lawrence's language of that colonial era was only slightly more moderate:

They are well built, cruel, hard looking fellows with not very dark skins. They claim to be the Lost Tribe of Israel and certainly they have a Semitic look about their nose and eyes.[7] I don't think it is the place to pass a lifetime in. All these Pathans are brought up to thieve, but in a camp like this there is less chance of losing one's kit than in Peshawar or Nowshera.

Lawrence was only among the Pathans for a month, during which they seem to have behaved themselves:

We'll be back in Nowshera now today week, after some strenuous sham fighting. The fighting may be sham, but the marching and running certainly is not. It is fine to watch the regiment extending out, moving like clockwork over ridges, dipping out of sight and then bursting into sight far away in an incredibly short time. It is a treat to see them drilling and marching, in their short rapid step. They twist their knees and strain ankles occasionally, but that is about all the work I have to do.

The enemy was a mild hazard compared with the mules:

We have hundreds of mules all round us and occasionally one breaks loose from its picketing and careers everywhere. You lie in bed at night and hear one galloping about everywhere and wonder when it is going to crash into your tent. The sound comes nearer and nearer and passes away with a great feeling of relief. They are apt to sit on your bed by the wall of your tent.

Lawrence's active service was one of the most pleasant it was possible to have. His illnesses during 1915–16 spared him from a posting on the Western Front and the fortuitous encounter with Bud Rose prevented him going to Mesopotamia. In 1918, he wrote, 'The sleepy old life goes on here the same as ever. Only the weather changes.' Lawrence was to have more than his fair share of bad luck during his life, but the three years in India were enriching and even enjoyable ones. He was well aware of how fortunate this posting was, as the quotes here from various letters show.

Thank goodness I became a doctor and nothing else. For one thing I probably shouldn't have been alive by this time in the war, which is always something to be thankful for.

Lawrence wrote home every single week from his voyage to India and during the three years he spent there. Above anything else, the letters highlight the exceptionally close and loving relationship he had with his family and especially with his mother. Only in a few of the more workaday letters do we get the sense that he is simply writing out of a sense of filial devotion. He wants to know every detail of how life is at home and records in detail his round of daily life: 'I like to have the homely news.' Although he was never actually homesick, he wrote longingly of outings they might make together on his return. He kept a photograph of his parents on his mantelpiece and put it in front of him when seated at his table writing home. When out on manoeuvres, he wrote his letters leaning on a biscuit tin.

This period of his life appears more like a set of gap years with some work experience. In one letter home, he suggested that

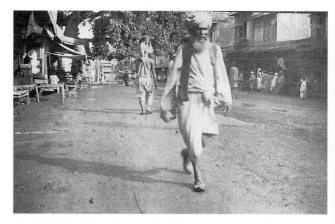

An old Pathan. From Lawrence's album.

his ambition was a chair in surgery, and in India he often felt frustrated that his medical career was not progressing very quickly and that much of his time was taken up with managing common infectious diseases as well as cases of plague and smallpox. 'My medical work is suffering woefully out here. I see no good cases and have got no books to read or study. Probably if I had, my energy wouldn't rise to it in this weather.' He dealt with a few chest cases. He longed for more experience in surgery and only worked on a few cases of adhesions, appendicitis and fractured limbs. There was also heat stroke, prickly heat and trench nephritis to attend to and he did not gain much satisfaction from simple first-aid work dealing largely with boils and whitlows.

He did get good experience in anaesthetics, as he gave two or three a week when doing hospital work. He also delivered a baby:

> I was wakened from a deep sleep one morning about 2 am – the sort of sleep in which you think: you have just gone to bed – to get an urgent chit from Smith, one of our assistant surgeons, saying that he had a private case which he thought required immediate Caesarean Section and would I come and do it at once. I thought this was rather a tall order for me, so I rushed inside to see if I could see anything about it in any of my books; but I could find nothing. So I drove along in the tonga trying to remember as much as I could about it and all the various steps of the operation. I got to the wretched native hovel where the patient was surrounded by native midwives and all the family friends groaning and lamenting. The favourite theory was that the child had got a hold of its mother's breast and thus could not be delivered. Fortunately the woman was unconscious and not worried by all this academic discussion and I found her to be in the dangerous fits of eclampsia, a disease of kidney origin of which you may have heard. I cleared the room quickly and found an operation unnecessary and managed to deliver the child with forceps quite easily, which was very lucky as I had never done it alone at the Coombe Hospital. After this, it was plain sailing and her fits stopped. That evening, however, she had a temp. of 106 F which we reduced with ice. Since then she has gradually got better and seems quite out of danger now, three days after. I put in for a good fee – 225 rupees (about £18) and it was paid up next day on the spot. All very satisfactory.

He then requested his mother to post him his textbook on midwifery.
Such hospital work as came his way he enjoyed:

> I have had a few more good operations lately at the hospital, two or three rather successful hernias and the other day I had a great time fishing for a halfpenny in a child's gullet. It came out all right in the end.

He benefited nicely from a visit to a private patient:

> I mentioned to you the rich patient I have in Peshawar who broke his leg in Nowshera some time ago. Well, I went to see him in Peshawar on Wednesday. The Khan Bahadur sent a motor car for me about 7.30 in the morning and I embarked at once, taking a friend Harvey with me. It was pretty hot by the time we reached Peshawar

city and we had an adventurous drive through its narrow streets to the house. The car didn't seem able to go slow and we hit a donkey on the nose and nearly ran over an old man before we reached our destination. The entrance was not prepossessing but when we got through a narrow alley we got into a palatial building, including private mosques and all sorts of fine houses. We were ushered into a large square room, very high and cold, surrounded by fine carved woodwork, in the intervals of which are little raised verandahs like rooms looking on to the big one. In one of these we had breakfast. Later my patient was lying in the middle of the large room, under a punkha, surrounded by crowds of relatives. These I cleared away and got to work. The patient is a very timid man, the sort that sighs and groans when I went near him and almost wept when I got a scissors to cut his bandage – and all this without suffering a scrap of pain, as he admitted himself. Well, I looked at his leg and found it healing nicely and in very good position. So I looked wise and said all was well. So ended the more professional part of the proceedings. After this I expressed a wish to see their underground rooms, so we descended into the bowels of the earth about 40 feet down to some rooms so cool and fresh that I nearly shivered with the contrast with above. And then tea was waiting Harvey and myself and we had a beautifully served tea with fine English silver and real lump sugar which I haven't seen anywhere else in India. And better still next came a fruit course with the choicest fruit I have had in the country, mangoes in perfection and passion fruit. I'm afraid we were rather gluttonous over the fruit, and Harvey felt squeamish when we got outside; but then he had just had malaria and we may be lenient in our judgement on this account. I next pocketed my 100 rupees (about £8) and had the motor at my disposal for the rest of the day. So I charged round the shops in the cantonment, buying socks, handkerchiefs and such-like things, some necessaries and some luxuries.

Lawrence related his experiences as a sanitary inspector:

I'm going to tell you the sort of work I have to do as Cantonment Medical Sanitary Officer. I set off on my bicycle to the Meat Market and there collect my minions, my white sanitary inspector, an old soldier; the bazaar/chaudri who sees that it is kept clean; and various subordinate knaves who carry my bicycle etc. After looking at the meat, about which, knowing nothing, I pretend to look wise and then we go to the vegetable market which is filled mostly with pumpkins and water melons and pomegranates and such-like uninviting things. Next we walk up the main shopping street with all the little shops – booths, most of them, you would say – and I poke about and see if anywhere the filth is so obvious that one must do something to stop it, usually imposing a fine which appeals to the native more than anything else. I poke into odd corners, liquor shops and see that the glasses etc are clean; into soda water factories to see that the water is boiled and filtered; into the ice factory. Then the other day I thought some of the native flour in one shop looked dark and adulterated, so I had it tested and found a large proportion of sand in it; so that chap was closed for a month and a fine imposed.

He reassured his mother: 'I am feeling well and not run down at all. There is no doubt that I am much stronger than I was five years ago.' But he makes frequent references to his snoozes and says that he feels sleepy but not tired. He complains of having a boil and also of having an ulcer on his leg that will not heal. He often comments on his thirst. It is tempting to make a *post hoc* diagnosis of the early onset of his diabetes, but so much can be explained by the slow pace of life and long periods of boredom in a hot, dusty country.

After the preceding years of study followed by several periods of illness and convalescence, he seized every opportunity not only for action, sport and adventure but also for self-improvement. He had been taught to ride at Aldershot in 1913, and developed a great love of riding and became a keen polo player. He hunted on horseback and also fished, climbed, played golf, hockey, badminton, tennis and went on numerous picnics and even did some tobogganing. He particularly enjoyed shooting duck and snipe, finding the latter particularly delicious. He had long holidays up in the hill station of Gulmarg and also around Srinagar, where he stayed on a houseboat. Kashmir was a favourite place:

The life here is the greatest change from Gulmarg. No engagements for golf, no dressing for dinner, no spick and span feeling. Instead I have been going about in a khaki shirt, old shorts, puttees and straw shoes in the most slovenly manner. I have been soothed by the tender stream, if not thrilled by its 'scaly denizens' as they would say in a newspaper. The stream is lovely; willows and green grass and rice fields make the sweetest of surroundings and we have dainty singing birds like at home, with wonderful kingfishers and golden oriels in addition, which flash

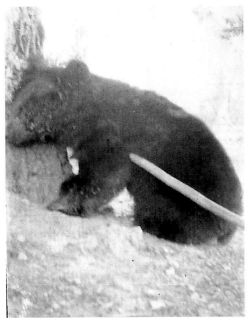

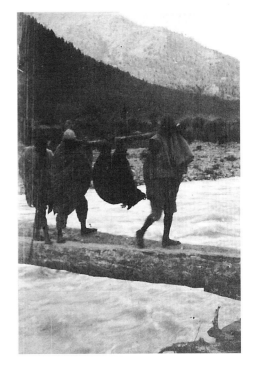

A bear hunt in the Sind Valley.

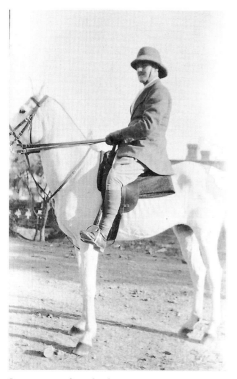

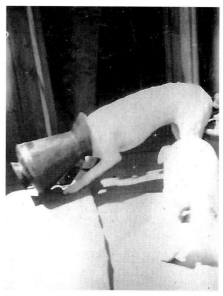

Lawrence's pet dog, Polly, in a spot of trouble with a pitcher.

Lawrence on horseback.

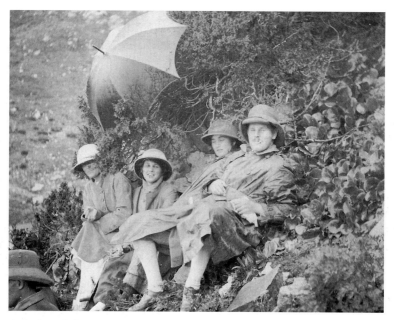

A picnic at Gulmarg.

brilliantly before one's eyes. And all around a magnificent circle of hills which I can never look at too much. My day has been fishing from 6 to 9 a.m., breakfast, a laze and sleep, tiffin and some reading, then fishing till dark and early to bed. My bearer does my cooking and most excellently. He is really a great treasure, quite a noble old man of about 45 as far as I can see; long may he stay with me.

Lawrence wrote the letters quoted in this and the preceding chapter between the ages of 23 and 26, and, in common with his generation – who had had to grow up very quickly with the onset of the War and the shocking loss of so many of their friends – he displays wisdom and maturity beyond his years and, apart from the odd outburst, does not take himself too seriously. Extensive quotes have been used here from an archive of over 150 letters. Apart from his own books that would be published later, it is the last time his voice can be heard in any sustained or developed way. Through these letters, we get to know him as a person in his own voice, and they reveal him as as a rounded character. One of his finest pieces of writing was produced when at camp in 1917:

The hour between sunset and dark seems to me far the finest in the life of the camp. Then only does one feel that camp can be a home rather than a restless and fleeting habitation. The day's work has slipped well behind us and the blind groping in the dark and the feeling of hostility and uncertainty in the country has not begun. The mules and horses have been brought into their lines and crowd snugly together in the friendliest of ways. They are cosy and tidy in their little blankets and have no food left to struggle and push for.
   And every evening about six the sunset clothes the whole landscape in beauty. The

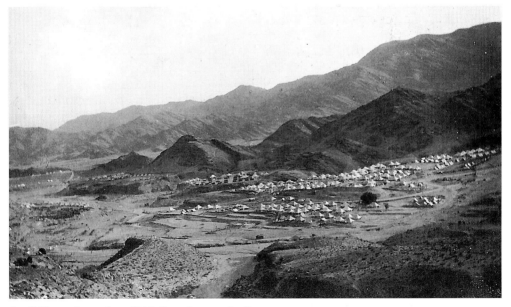

Lundi Khana Camp, June 1919. From Lawrence's album

west side of the camp is higher than the rest and overlooks a flat plain stretching to the lower hills. Here one or two of us collect – and I never miss it, to watch the sun setting behind the distant mountains. Their bold and jagged outlines show up strikingly against the glowing colours of the sky and such is the effect of the light that the skyline of every ridge seemed crowned by a ribbon of silver of extraordinary brightness. The near slope of the hills is misty in purple and blues which change to sable and black as the light creeps slowly out of the sky. And now the wire defences are put out for the night and no one may stir from our little home of some hundreds of yards in area till another day comes to bore or delight us, as the case may be.

And then I stroll back to my tent where the lamp is waiting to welcome me and the native boy to help the sahib to change. The bath is hot, but not much deeper than an inch and is carried out in the back parlour of the tent where it is impossible to move or turn without bringing down showers of dust from the walls. And even in my bed-sitting-room, it is impossible to stand straight without ruffling my hair or without my boy knocking his turban off – and he must never be bare-headed nor even appear with his shoes on in the presence of his sahib. My tables and wardrobes are made out of old boxes and all kinds of things to wear are suspended on ropes slung across the tent like drying ropes.

And now comes the time I like best of the whole day when one tastes the atmosphere of camp life to its full and the wonderful contrast of east and west which a camp containing both British and native troops always presents. I go on to a path which is the main thoroughfare of the camp and watch the life there. It is the half-hour before Mess when it is not unpleasantly dark enough to make one stumble over tent pegs and into holes and strain one's eyes to see anything. On one side is the coffee shop and the beer shop, cheek by jowl, with a crowd of men gathered in the light by the counter, chatting and joking and spending their pay on their stomachs. Others are carrying away meat pies and mugs of beer to their tents and one gets a glimpse of an open door of cosy parties of men playing cards or reading old magazines or papers. The sentries are posted all round the camp and can be heard challenging occasionally, though the tread of their feet is muffled in the sand … all this is western enough.

On the other side of the road the picture is of the unchanging east. Round tiny fires made of scraps of wood, groups of native sepoys are squatting on their haunches. They are wrapped in their whitish cloth with everything but their noses covered and are chattering away in a strange musical language, making an occasional gesture with a bony black hand or stretching it out to warm at the meagre blaze. They are the mysterious crawling figures which one sees all over India, by the roadside, in the booths of the bazaar, in the compounds of bungalows. Some of them are cooking queer messes on their brass dishes, filling the air with over-powering and horrible smells of garlic and some special kind of fat.

Suddenly one notices that the light is replaced by blackness and that it is cold, and very glad I am to slip into the Mess to hot soup and a five-course dinner, to be followed by chatting and perhaps a game of bridge. Then I read myself to sleep in bed, which usually takes about five minutes and know nothing till morning, unless I am wakened by a burst of barking from the pariah dogs of a native village about half a mile away. Goodnight. RDL

Although news of the Armistice reached him quickly enough, it was a year before he returned home via Alexandria in Egypt, where he worked at the Ras el Jin Military Hospital and later contracted dysentery. He was discharged as an Officer in the RAMC Reserve and declared unfit to continue further military service, which pleased him a lot. He returned home around 27 October 1919 and sped north for the long-awaited reunion with his family.

The letters end here, leaving a silence where his voice had been so clear for three years.

References

1. The *Miltiades* was a 6793 gross-ton ship, length 455 ft × beam 55.1 ft, clipper bows, one funnel, two masts, twin-screw, speed 15 knots, accommodation considered luxurious for 89 First Class and 158 Third Class passengers. Completed in October 1903 by Alex Stephen & Sons, Glasgow, for the Aberdeen Line, she started her maiden voyage from London for Cape Town, Melbourne and Sydney on 3 November 1903. In 1912, she was rebuilt to 7817 tons and lengthened to 504 ft and a second funnel was added. Accommodation was increased to 150 First Class and 170 Third Class. Taken up for trooping duties in 1915, she resumed commercial service on 4 June 1920, but started her last Australia voyage on 20 November 1920. Purchased by the Royal Mail Steam Packet Co. and renamed *Orcana*, she was transferred to the Pacific Steam Navigation Co. in 1922 for their 'Round South America' service. However, she proved too expensive to operate and the second voyage was cancelled. In 1923, she was laid up at Liverpool and later at Dartmouth, and in 1924 she was towed to Holland and scrapped. (Details from Haws D. *Merchant Fleets*, Volume 17: Aberdeen and Commonwealth Lines. Hereford: TCL Publications, 1989.)
2. *Kinfaun's Castle* was built in 1899, became a Union Castle mail ship in 1900 and was scrapped in 1927.
3. Woodward DR. *The Middle East during World War One*. www.bbc.co.uk/history/worldwars/wwone/middle_east_01.shtml
4. *Kashmiri Song* is a song by Amy Woodforde-Finden based on a poem by Laurence Hope, pseudonym of Adela Florence Nicolson: 'Pale hands I loved beside the Shalimar,/Where are you now? Who lies beneath your spell?/ Whom do you lead on Rapture's roadway, far,/Before you agonise them in farewell?'
5. He is referring to the scar tissue from recent operations.
6. The Pathans are now referred to as Pashtuns and are the world's largest autonomous tribal society. They are for the most part Sunni Muslims, religiously conservative and proud of their early conversion to Islam. They follow a very strict code of behaviour with emphasis on hospitality, honour, revenge and complete submission of the vanquished. (Singh S, Brown L, Clammer P et al. *Pakistan and the Karakoram Highway*, 7th edn. London: Lonely Planet Publications, 2008.)
7. This is probably not the case, since their language has no roots in common. However, it is likely that some were descended from the remnants of Alexander the Great's invading army. (Personal communication from Dr NJ Spivey, University of Cambridge.)

CHAPTER 5

Pioneering the Use of Insulin and Setting up a Diabetes Service: 1923–1934

On his return from India, Lawrence steamed north to be reunited with his family in Aberdeen and to enjoy all the homely things he had missed so much in his three years abroad. He also managed to satisfy his longing for trout fishing by 'poaching two beauties (3–4 lbs) in the river Don'.

He may well have stayed on in Aberdeen to celebrate Christmas and his father's birthday before returning to London to find a job and to study for the second part of his FRCS. Most hospitals were giving priority to their own students, but, as described in Chapter 1, he managed to secure an appointment as second House Surgeon in the Casualty Department of King's College Hospital, London SE5, probably in January 1920.

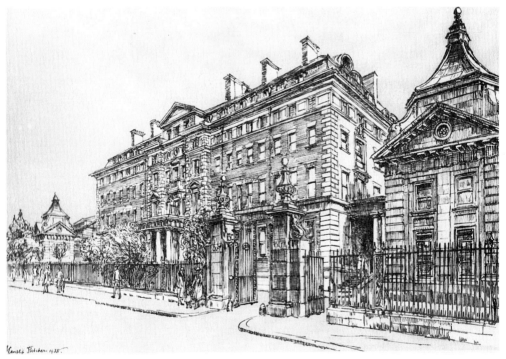

King's College Hospital, by Hanslip Fletcher (1874–1955).

This gave him wide and varied experience, but it was exhausting work. His bedroom was some distance away from Casualty (in one note, he states it was four miles, and another 400 yards). When the emergency bell rang, he would leap out of bed, throw on his gym shoes and sprint to Casualty, arriving hot and breathless – not at all in a fit state to attend to serious casualties. His solution was to get a bike with a loud bell that enabled him to race through the corridors and appear in a more befitting way for work, but unfortunately the bell woke the Matron, who was clearly a zealous pioneer of the Health and Safety movement and did not approve of a young doctor careering through the corridors on a bike waking everyone en route. She complained to the authorities, and so it was back to the gym shoes and the sprinting.

His work was clearly satisfactory, for after six months of Casualty work, he was told he could apply for any job he wanted at King's, as if he were a King's man. He was appointed assistant surgeon in the Ear, Nose and Throat Department and threw himself into his new work with enthusiasm and energy while enjoying a busy social and sporting life. Those frustrating wartime years of waiting in a distant corner of the Empire were behind him and he was on the way to achieving a career in surgery. During this time, he played hockey and tennis for the hospital and worked regularly until 1 am. The onset of his diabetes and his subsequent return home has been told in Chapter 1.

Articles in newspapers in 1923 led the public to believe that insulin was a cure and before-and-after photographs of children who had been resurrected offered dramatic evidence of its power. The most famous are those of Kansas professor of medicine Ralph Major's patient Billy Leroy in the June 1923 *Journal of the American Medical Association*. At the time of the first picture, this three-year-old boy had had diabetes for two years and weighed only 6.8 kg. After three months, his weight had increased to 13.6 kg and his urine was sugar-free on a regimen of 55 g carbohydrate and 25 units of insulin daily.[1]

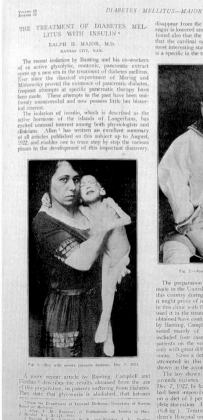
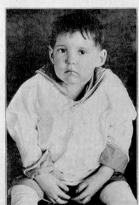

Billy Leroy before and after his treatment with insulin. Reproduced by permission, Wellcome Trust.

The practice of medicine in the 1920s was very different from today. The forte of hospital physicians was diagnosis and most illnesses they dealt with ran their natural course, either to recovery or to death. The only effective drugs in their armamentarium were morphine, thyroid extract, phenobarbitone, digitalis, laxatives and sedatives. Apart from myxoedema, easily controlled by thyroid extract, the only chronic disease that needed continuous treatment and monitoring was diabetes, treated by diet.

Insulin was totally different to anything in the pharmacopoeia. For one thing it had to be given by injection. For another, unlike previous so-called diabetes treatments, it was extremely potent, with potentially dangerous side effects. In 1923, in the *BMJ*, the Professor of Medicine at St Thomas', Hugh Maclean, warned that 'Every medical man employing insulin should be thoroughly impressed with the fact that he is using a powerful and dangerous, though easily controlled, remedy, and that any neglect on his part may end in disaster.'[2]

Apart from the dangers, there were many other questions that Lawrence and his fellow pioneers needed to answer, including the following:

- Could patients inject themselves and how should they be taught to do it?
- Was diabetes progressive and, if not, would insulin rest the pancreas enough for regeneration to take place?
- What level of blood sugar should be aimed for and were regular blood sugar measurements necessary?
- Could the old dietary restrictions be abandoned?
- How dangerous was hypoglycaemia?
- Could insulin treatment be started and supervised by general practitioners (GPs)?

These questions preoccupied Lawrence for the next decade, and he had an advantage over other diabetes specialists in that he could and did experiment on himself. He was an inpatient at King's from May to October 1923, during which time his weight increased by 17 lb (7.71 kg). As his health improved, so did his activity, and the records show that he was out dancing twice in a week (once until 4 am), busy on his exercise machine and also playing tennis.

Injections

The first problem with the new treatment was injections. Many, if not most, physicians doubted whether ordinary patients could be taught to self-inject – even though they knew that rich morphine addicts did. In his first paper on insulin, in 1923, Joslin remarked that 'intelligent patients can be taught the use of diet and insulin in a week', while, for Lawrence, 'one minute's practical demonstration of an injection will teach a patient more than pages of writing [since] all doctors and, indeed, many patients are quite familiar with hypodermic injections'. Lawrence claimed that few patients had difficulties after the first week and that 'the initial repugnance that many patients feel to daily injections soon gives way to the indifference of an easy habit'. He advised that injections could be given anywhere the skin was loose, such as the thighs, abdomen and lower chest. In 1925, he specifically advised against using the calves, although this seems to be a case of 'do as I say, not as I do', since we know that he injected not only into his calves but also through his clothes.

The metal syringes with leather plungers in use before the First World War had been replaced by all-glass French-made Luer syringes and many doctors advised boiling them before each injection, which led to many breakages and consequent expense. Lawrence wrote that 'all my patients keep their syringes in methylated spirit or absolute alcohol and never sterilize them by boiling or strong antiseptics. In this way trouble is minimised, and not a single abscess or infection of any kind has occurred in patients of all classes and conditions.' Needles did have to be resharpened regularly with a stone.

Early insulin preparations were relatively impure, some more so than others, and often caused local swelling and irritation. Thus, in July 1923 when Lawrence changed from American to British insulin, he noted that the injections caused more marked local reactions. He summarized the types of reactions in a paper in the *Lancet* in 1925 in which he was the first illustrative case.[3] He returned to the subject in 1928 in a paper in which he reported the results of microscopic examination of biopsies of his own injection sites.[4]

Another difficulty in 1923–24 was that the potency of insulin varied from batch to batch, which was a problem for those such as Lawrence who were attempting close control of their blood sugar levels. Lawrence tested the strength of new batches on himself and his laboratory assistant H. R. Millar, who also had diabetes. In 1925, with G. A. Harrison and H. P. Marks from the Biological Standards Department of the Medical Research Council (MRC), he wrote a paper that showed that laboratory measurement of the strength of insulin using rabbits correlated well with the time-consuming clinical measurements.[5]

Progression of the disease and the possibility of regeneration

The idea that resting the pancreas with insulin might lead to regeneration of the islet cells was not just wishful thinking. Kidneys could recover after acute glomerulonephritis and the lungs after lobar pneumonia, so why not the pancreas? In 1923, none other than Banting had written that, 'Regardless of the severity of the disease it has been found that by carefully adjusting the diet and the dose of insulin, all patients may be maintained sugar free. Since this is possible, it is to be strongly advocated because we have abundant evidence for the belief that there is regeneration of the islet cells of the pancreas when the strain thrown upon them by a high blood sugar is relieved.'[6]

Lawrence also hoped that a cure might be possible and in his Banting Memorial Lecture in 1949 wrote that 'In 1923 it seemed possible that one might cure diabetes or recreate pancreatic function by keeping the blood-sugar normal, or below normal, for a long time. For six months, therefore, I lived on a very low diet (16 g. carbohydrate, 70 g. protein, 100 g. fat), with all the insulin I could stand, only 15 units a day (8 and 7). After 6 months of this weary existence, I ate more and my requirements rose to 40 units; I became if not fighting, at least playing, fit.'[7]

In fact, the records show that this experiment lasted two weeks rather than six months! He may have confused his own experience with an experiment by his erstwhile colleague Geoffrey Harrison, who, in 1925 at Great Ormond Street Hospital, studied five patients, aged 32–47, who were kept on a fixed diet for 46–83 weeks, with their insulin dose being adjusted to maintain a normal blood sugar. The dose often had to be reduced in the first few days, but there was no evidence of even a partial remission thereafter and most needed slightly more insulin at the end of the experimental period (partly because all had put on weight).[8]

Blood sugar levels and their measurement

After a few weeks on insulin, patients recovered their health and strength even without achieving normal blood sugar levels, which raised the question of whether the success of treatment should be determined by clinical endpoints such as vigour and weight or biochemical ones such as absence of sugar in the urine and normal blood sugars. Chapters by George Graham of Bart's and Edward Poulton (1883–1939) of Guy's in two popular British medical textbooks recommended that the urine should always be sugar-free and the fasting blood sugar between 4.4 and 6.7 mmol/L.[9] Most American physicians also believed in the goal of physiological normality, the most uncompromising being Joslin, who, in the 1928 edition of his textbook, wrote:

> Glycosuria is not only tolerated but encouraged by several physicians highly skilled in the treatment of diabetes. Even 20 grams of glucose are allowed in the urine by design. To this plan of treatment I am emphatically opposed ... success in the treatment of diabetic children lies in keeping their urine sugar-free. If sugar appears, a penalty follows.

The penalty was not blindness or kidney failure, because for 15 years after the discovery of insulin these only affected middle-aged patients. Joslin probably meant susceptibility to infection. Unfortunately, physiological normality was an impossible ideal for most patients with the tools they had at their disposal. In 1925, in the first edition of his patient handbook, *The Diabetic Life*, Lawrence wrote that 'the attempt to keep the blood sugar constantly normal may be ideal in theory but in practice it is very difficult to achieve and makes the diabetic life unnecessarily hard without adequate benefit'.[10]

Insulin caused blood sugar to fall

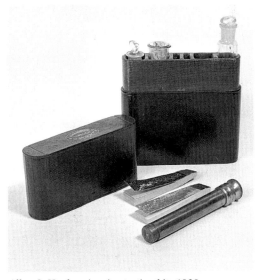

Allen & Hanbury's urine testing kit, 1920s.

rapidly, with urine sugar levels lagging behind. In hospital, insulin treatment was monitored by blood tests, and a *Lancet* editorial in 1923 ended by saying, 'but when he leaves [hospital] matters are very different. His medical adviser can administer the daily dose of insulin but what about the blood sugar determinations?'[11] By 1923, micro-methods had been developed that meant that blood sugar could be measured from a finger prick by those who had a laboratory and the necessary technical skills. Kits were marketed with which (in theory) GPs or patients could measure blood sugar. In response to an advertisement in the *BMJ* for Maclean's blood sugar measuring kit, one indignant GP wrote that it needed 'Fifteen special pieces of apparatus and six special solutions. It requires a room, or at least a bench, set apart for its use. It takes one hour to carry the test through, and experimental errors due to want of practice in the use of capillary tubes make it essential to perform more than one estimation in order to obtain a reliable result.'[12]

Predictably, he recommended sticking to quantitative urine tests with Fehling's

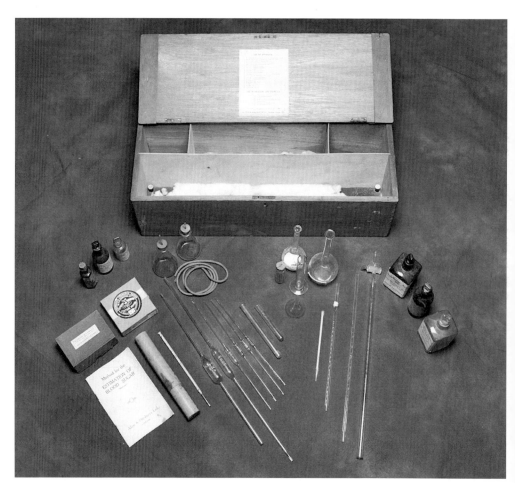

Allen & Hanbury's blood sugar equipment using Maclean's method – probably dated 1929 – with all the chemicals and glassware intact.

solution. Thus, it came to be accepted that blood sugar would be measured at clinic visits but that the main form of monitoring would be urine tests. By no means all physicians believed that patients should be encouraged or would be able to check their own condition with urine testing. For those who were judged suitable, the most commonly used test was Benedict's, in which the urine was boiled with a copper solution. If there was no sugar, the solution remained blue, while if there was a lot, it turned brick-red. Lawrence explained the technique in *The Diabetic Life* in plain English as follows:

Put 8 drops of urine in a clean test-tube. Add 1 inch (1 teaspoonful) of blue solution. Shake test-tube. Stand the test-tube in a small pan of boiling water and boil for five minutes; or boil in spirit or gas flame for two minutes. Then take out the test-tube. If the fluid remains clear and blue, no sugar is present; if the fluid turns slightly green and a greyish sediment appears at the bottom of the tube, there is still no sugar present. If the solution goes green and there is a yellow deposit after standing for ten minutes, a little sugar is present. If the solution goes yellow, a considerable amount of sugar is present. If the solution goes brown or red, very heavy amounts of sugar are present. There is also very heavy sugar present if brown or red tests turns to a dirty green (olive) colour, which some patients mistake for the light green trace of sugar.

Lest the reader might have thought this rather complicated, Lawrence added, 'When you have been shown a few tests you will find urine testing quite simple.'

Diet

When insulin was first marketed in April 1923, 100 units cost 25s 0d, but a year later this had fallen to 6s 8d. To save money and avoid wasting precious insulin, it was then standard practice to continue the very-low-carbohydrate pre-insulin diet. As late as 1926, patients under George Graham at Bart's were given a preliminary fast 'to emphasize to them the seriousness of their disease'. Only if the carbohydrate could not be raised to 40–50 g per day without causing glycosuria was insulin started. Lawrence thoroughly disapproved of this approach, and in the first edition of *The Diabetic Life* (1925) wrote:[13]

Starvation has some definite drawbacks, some obvious, others less recognised. Firstly, it is a dreaded and disagreeable way of de-sugarising a patient and may lead to an unnecessary loss of weight and strength which it may be difficult to recover. ... some authorities still commence treatment with starvation and a slowly progressive diet, instead of the basal diet advocated here. The process is slow and tedious and completely interrupts the patient's ordinary life. Insulin is withheld until the last possible moment.

In the pre-insulin era diet had meant restriction of food intake. Now, as Lawrence quickly realized, it meant balancing the dose of insulin with the appropriate amount of carbohydrate. His view was that insulin was easier to alter than diet, so he taught that the diet should be as constant as possible. He wrote:

> *Everyone recognises that the most difficult part of the battle, both for the doctor and for the patient, is not the insulin but the quantitative diet necessary in severe cases. A diet should be accurate and simple and yet permit a variety to suit all tastes and purses. If the diet is accurate and simple yet rigid, it often defeats its own object by the patient getting tired of the monotony.*

Teaching the diet was a problem. In America, elite institutions such as Joslin's clinic in Boston and the Mayo Clinic held classes. From 1913, at the private Duff House Sanatorium in Banff, Scotland, Dr E. L. (later Sir Edmund) Spriggs (1871–1949) had organized sessions that included a class by the diet nurse and a demonstration of urine testing by laboratory staff. Spriggs produced what must have been one of the first patient-orientated books, *A Manual of Diet on Diabetes for Patients at Duff House* which ran to 20 chapters, including one on 'special gardening'. At the Medical Society of London in 1921, Spriggs suggested that every hospital should organize such classes for in- and outpatients, since 'the expense would be trifling and the benefits great'. It seems likely that this fell on deaf ears because most voluntary hospitals would not have had the space, staff or funds to run classes for patients, most of whom were implicitly regarded as uneducable.

In plain terms, Lawrence stated that if he could not understand calories, how on earth could one expect the little old ladies and men of Camberwell to understand them? His patients, he said, ate food not calories. His solution was the line ration diet.[14] Food items on the chart were coloured black or red, and one black portion plus one red was equal to one line ration. Each black portion had 10 g carbohydrate and each red portion 7.5 g protein and 9 g fat. At first, the number of red portions had to be equal to the number of black portions, but gradually, as confidence in carbohydrate grew, the line diet was modified to increase the number of black portions and to reduce the dependence on fat as a source of calories. The reason for the protein and fat values of the red portion was that 10 red portions provided the average amount of protein and fat in the average British diet of the time. The number of lines to be prescribed per day was obtained by dividing the person's weight in pounds by 16, or, as Lawrence wrote, '16.5 is more exact'. The scheme is shown on the next page.

Somewhat optimistically Lawrence thought that patients could grasp the scheme in two minutes, with the only irksome aspect being accurate weighing of the food, for which he recommended a letter scales costing four or five shillings, although for those with more money confectioner's scales were better.

The diabetic diet was advantageous where the bowels were concerned. In response to a paper in the *BMJ* in 1926 by Colonel (later Sir) Robert McCarrison (1878–1960), director of nutritional research for the Indian Medical Service, extolling the virtues of a high-fibre diet of unrefined food,[15] Lawrence wrote to say that the diabetic diet was similar. He recalled that one of his patients, 'who is allowed 15 grams of carbohydrate for breakfast insists on taking it all as vegetables, and starts the day with 18 oz. of cabbage along with his bacon and egg! This is as

The 'line ration' diet scheme

ONE BLACK PORTION ADDED TO ONE TINTED PORTION = ONE LINE RATION	
Black portions (carbohydrate foods: containing sugar or starch): 10 g carbohydrate	Red portions (protein and fat): 7½ g protein and 9 g fat
Rice, sago, tapioca (raw)	One egg
Biscuit, toast or breakfast cereals; ½ flour, oatmeal, macaroni (all dry); jam or marmalade	Bacon or ham (both lean) 1 oz
Bread (all kinds)	Kidney 1¼ oz and fat ¼ oz
Potato, peas or beans (dried or 2 oz tinned); banana or grapes; dried apricots (stewed)	Liver 1 oz. and fat ¼ oz
Parsnips; ripe greengages; prunes (stewed) 3 oz	Tongue (tinned or fresh) 1 oz.
Raw apple, pear, cherries, gooseberries, plums, damsons, orange (skinned); young peas or beetroot 4 oz	Tripe or sweetbreads 1¼ oz and fat ¼ oz
Peach or apricot or black currants (ripe); greengages (stewed); broad beans 5 oz	Lean beef or veal 1 oz and fat ¼ oz
Strawberries; stewed pears, damsons or plums 6 oz	Lean lamb or mutton 1 oz and fat ¼ oz
Milk (also contains 1 Red); black currants (stewed); raspberries or melon (ripe) 7 oz	Lean pork 1 oz
*Apples or cherries (stewed); carrots or leeks 8 oz	Chicken or pigeon 1 oz. and fat ¼ oz
*Jerusalem artichokes; loganberries; blackberries (stewed) 10 oz	Duck 1 oz
*Grapefruit (in skin); tomatoes; red currants 12 oz	Pheasant, grouse or partridge ¾ oz and fat ¼ oz
*Onions, turnips or radishes 14 oz	Rabbit or hare ¾ oz and fat ¼ oz
Half portions of these are usually enough. *Negligible starch content in average helpings of:* Asparagus, green artichokes, French beans, Brussels sprouts, cabbage, cauliflower, celery, cranberries, cress, cucumber, egg plant, endive, stewing gooseberries, greens, horseradish, lemons, lettuce, marrow, mushrooms, radishes, rhubarb, salsify, scarlet runners, seakale, spinach	Crab or lobster 1¼ oz and fat ¼ oz
	Herring 1 oz and fat ¼ oz
	Kipper 1 oz and fat ¼ oz
	Salmon 1 oz and fat ¼ oz
	Sardines 1 oz
	White fish (all kinds) 1¼ oz and fat ¼ oz
	Cheese ¾ oz
	Milk 7 oz (also contains 1 Black)
Extras of no food value: Tea, coffee, soda water, Bovril, Oxo, etc., ordinary condiments and flavourings	Fats are meat fats, suet, dripping, butter, margarine, olive oil; thick cream in twice the amount stated for other fats

close an approximation to the pre-agricultural diet of primitive man ... as modern man is ever likely to tolerate. I have never seen the constipation of a lifetime able to withstand such a diet.'[16]

By 1927, when insulin was freely available and cost less than 2s per 100 units, many were still prescribing very low-carbohydrate diets. At the British Medical Association Annual Meeting that year, Lawrence remembered that 'MacLean[17] and Petrén[18] were still using very low carbohydrate diets (20–30 grams), and the latter, minimal carbohydrate and protein with very high fat – 200 grams or more. A few workers in this country had raised the carbohydrate to from 50 to 100 grams, but seldom higher, and fat still predominated as the calorie producer in the diabetic diet.'[19]

From 1926, several North American physicians, including Rawle Geyelin (1883–1942) of the New York Presbyterian Hospital,[20] William Sansum (1880–1948) of Santa Barbara[21] and Israel Rabinowitch (1890–1983) of Montreal,[22] promoted what they saw as the advantages of high-carbohydrate diets. Among these were that they increased the relative effectiveness of insulin and were more palatable and cheaper. Nevertheless, many physicians resisted because it seemed intuitively that more insulin would be needed and there was also concern that patients were not trustworthy and that, if given an inch, would take a mile. Lawrence reviewed these studies in the *BMJ* in 1932, the year in which he was elected FRCP.[23] In the preamble, he wrote that:

> I should like to emphasize that, as diabetics can be kept well on all three types of diet [low-, moderate- and high-carbohydrate], a most important criterion of the success of their treatment is their personal comfort and happiness. We must satisfy the patient, and, if we can, minimize the troubles of dieting and weighing and calculating grams of carbohydrate, protein, and fat, and total calories. We must try for the comfort of the patient to keep down the number of injections to two and for the sake of expense the total of units per day.

He had tried free diets in which patients ate what they pleased and had found that enormous doses of insulin were necessary. He had also watched the effect of uncontrolled diets in a few unrestrainable patients and had 'seen the difficulties'. He did not specify what the difficulties were, but others had found that weight gain was one consequence. 'In conclusion', Lawrence wrote, 'I believe that many types and variations of diet work well so long as adequate insulin is given. To obtain the most satisfactory results the treatment can and should be modified from case to case to suit the comfort and habits of the patient.'

This sort of individualization of treatment was not practised by most diabetes specialists at the time. It was, of course, by Lawrence in managing his own diabetes; if he wanted to eat something extra, say in a restaurant, he simply gave an extra shot of insulin.

Hypoglycaemia

Before the discovery of insulin, the concept of hypoglycaemia was foreign to physicians and physiologists. The only way to make an animal hypoglycaemic was to remove or poison its liver, and the symptoms were impossible to distinguish from the effects of surgery or the poisons. In a paper in the 1922 *Journal of Metabolic Research*, not published until May 1923, the Toronto physicians described the amazing variety of symptoms caused by low blood sugar:[24]

> *The initial symptom may be a feeling of nervousness or tremulousness, sometimes a feeling of excessive hunger, at other times a feeling of weakness or a sense of goneness. The level at which a patient becomes aware of the fall in blood sugar is fairly constant for that individual, although this is not always the case … [as the blood sugar falls further] … the feeling of nervousness may become definite anxiety, excitement or even emotional upset. The feeling of tremulousness is possibly a form of incoordination. Patients have shown a loss of power to perform fine movements with their fingers … Much more severe manifestations are observed with further lowering of the blood sugar. Marked excitement, emotional instability, sensory and motor aphasia, dysarthria, delirium, disorientation, confusion have all been seen.*

As far as we know, Lawrence did not get any of the more dramatic manifestations during his first years on insulin, but he found that exercise needed careful adjustments to avoid hypoglycaemia. In 1924, he tried skiing for the first time since using insulin and this:

> *required skilful adjustments, both for climbing up and for getting up from falling down into deep snow – equally strenuous. On skiing days I reduced the morning insulin from 15 to 10 units, had an extra roll for breakfast and filled two rolls with honey or black cherry jam to eat after climbing; I also took the usual packed lunch and, of course, sugar in every pocket. On return to the hotel after this very strenuous day, I often felt not only exhausted but very hungry and slightly thirsty, obviously getting diabetic with the reduced morning dose quite exhausted: so I often took an extra small injection (6–10 units) before a fairly normal tea – coffee usually, with a few sandwiches and a cream cake or two, bathed and slept, and took a much reduced dose before dinner, as some of the tea-time dose was still active. With this and other slight modifications, I became as fit and capable of strenuous activity as anybody.*

In 1926, he published a paper 'Effect of exercise on insulin action'.[25] Two cases were described, both young men who were 'skilful and careful dietitians and keen observers of their own condition'. Case 1, whom we assume to be Lawrence, is described in great detail in relation to the effect of his weekend tennis and a strenuous three-week holiday. Case 2, a gardener, did hard physical work every day and needed half the amount of insulin taken by the more sedentary Lawrence. Case 1 did an experiment on himself in which he took strenuous exercise that caused his blood sugar to fall precipitously from 250 to 50 mg/dL (13.9 to 2.8 mmol/L) over 2½ hours, compared with a gradual fall to 180 mg/dL (10 mmol/L) when no exercise was taken. After the strenuous exercise, hypoglycaemia recurred within 2 hours of taking glucose, which Lawrence correctly surmised was due to depletion of carbohydrate stores.

Time. Minutes.	A. Insulin + Exercise.	B. Insulin, no Exercise.
2 p.m.	240 Insulin 10 units	254 Insulin 10 units
20	245	–
30	–	242
45	219	–
60	175	239
90	116	230
120	73*	211
150 4.30 p.m.	51*	181

The effect of 10 units of insulin on diabetic blood sugar. A, with exercise; B, no exercise.
* Symptoms of hypoglycaemia

Effect of exercise on insulin action: BMJ *10 April 1926.*[24]

Could insulin treatment be started and supervised by GPs?

The assertions of both Lawrence and Joslin about the simplicity of treatment raised the question of insulin use by GPs. This was debated at the Annual Meeting of the British Medical Association in September 1923 and answered by Banting, as a former surgeon, in typically forthright terms:[26]

> *When a patient was discharged from hospital in Toronto a long detailed letter was sent to the family physician but by the time the patient left hospital he was thoroughly au fait with the routine … There was no reason why diabetic patients should not be treated as well by the general practitioner as by the specialist.*

Toronto General Hospital began courses for family physicians in early 1923 and several large American hospitals quickly followed suit. The response of English physicians seems to have been ambivalent in that in their writings they encouraged GPs to use insulin, but there is no indication that they organized courses where GPs could learn the practical aspects. Also, because of the way the British system was organized, there was a positive incentive for physicians to guard their skills and income. Another barrier was that the level of sophistication in general practice in England at the time was low; until 1950, when the preregistration year was instituted, a student could put up his plate as a GP the day after qualifying and never have any further education. Another thing the experts ignored was that diabetes in the under-40s was sufficiently rare that a GP might never (knowingly) see a case during their career. After a lecture on insulin by a London physician, the average GP might well have agreed with a Dr R. Sanderson, who at a meeting in

Brighton suggested that 'whatever may be the benefits conferred on the diabetic by insulin, there seemed little doubt that it bade fair to bring many practitioners to a premature grave so multitudinous, bewildering and worrying were the problems involved'.[27]

Diabetic clinics

It thus became accepted that those with diabetes who needed insulin would be looked after by hospitals. However, the way the healthcare system was organized in Britain was not conducive to the management of this new chronic disease. Hospital physicians prided themselves on being generalists and, if not actively hostile to special clinics, did not support them.

The first diabetic clinic in Britain was started in Edinburgh in 1924 by David Murray Lyon (1888–1956). The *Lancet,* commenting on the special clinics that had been started in Edinburgh (tuberculosis and lupus were the other two), approved because[28]

The advantage of this organised method of treating patients suffering from diseases requiring lengthy treatment lies in ensuring a concentrated study of the special disease, and in obtaining correct and persistent treatment, which is so essential for satisfactory results. The amount of time and labour saved is very considerable, the collecting of statistics is greatly facilitated, opportunities for mass experiments are afforded, and from the point of view of teaching the method offers many advantages. From the economic and social standpoint it would seem to provide the solution to the problem of dealing with chronic disease.

Nevertheless, diabetic clinics were the exception rather than the rule for the next 20 years; those who could afford it were seen privately, while ordinary patients were followed up in general medical clinics that were totally unsuitable for education or long-term follow-up. Gladys Wauchope (1889–1966), who herself developed diabetes in 1926, remembered that in 1920, when she was clinical assistant to Medical Outpatients at the London Hospital, the session lasted from 1 pm to 7 pm. Large numbers of patients attended, most of whom had come for 'Rep Mist' (repeat the mixture). She set up the first diabetic clinic in Brighton in 1934 and soon found that up to a hundred patients would attend in 2½ hours to be seen by two or three doctors. Laconically, she commented that 'one acquires a knack of working fast without appearing to hurry.'[29]

In 1924, Lawrence virtually lived in the laboratory, learning a great deal about biochemistry. He is quoted as saying that he had 'a demon passion for work' and seldom did a day go by when he did not undertake an experiment on himself, on a patient or on an animal. He recorded that, each week, more insulin became available and that more diabetics were put on it, so there was a great and growing crowd in the laboratory and not much room for any general biochemistry. 'Nothing but diabetics sitting about waiting to have blood tests. An awful shambles.' Because he did not have any beds, patients had perforce to be treated as outpatients. He wrote, 'we are in the habit of treating practically all newly diagnosed patients from the start as outpatients, with the exception of cases of coma, children under 16, those who live at too great a distance to attend hospital daily and the intensely stupid patients.' Teaching of diet and insulin therapy became so difficult that a side room of a ward was set aside and equipped by a generous gift from a wealthy Australian diabetic. A full-time sister was appointed to take charge of the diet kitchen. She fed the patients and taught them about diets and injections, so a new diabetic department began to develop, albeit in rather a piecemeal way. A full-time special staff nurse was employed. By 1928, at least 500 diabetic patients were attending the Outpatient Department. In the following year, an additional nurse was employed in the diabetic kitchen.

As the numbers at King's increased, with 1292 patients in 1929, 2069 in 1931 and 2472 in 1933, the opportunity was taken ('bagged') to move the clinic. At a meeting of the Committee of Management on 6 April 1933, it was agreed that a vacated museum be used for diabetes. At the same meeting, the famous letter from Lawrence's patient and friend, the author H. G. Wells to *The Times* was authorized. This letter was published on 19 April 1933 and described the cramped space for patients and laboratory equipment and appealed for £700–£800 for

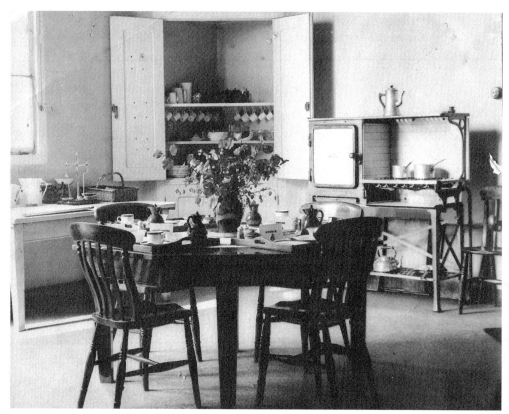

Diet kitchen at King's, 1920s. Weighing and measuring equipment is on the shelf at the back.

much needed space, light, ventilation and material. Wells wrote, 'I suggest that it would be a becoming thing for the elect class of grateful diabetics to whom I appeal to tax themselves for the benefit of our cult.' A donation of £20 each was suggested and 'the participation of friendly non-diabetics will rouse no resentment'. On 6 June 1933, £316 from the H. G. Wells Diabetic Fund allowed structural work on the clinic to proceed, and on 3 October a total of £800 was reached with a gift of £324 from a William Chapman of Cape Town. This became the Outpatient Department for the next 40 years. A waiting room was created to seat 100 patients, and this soon became the average attendance for the three main clinics of the week. The clinic itself was an open space with six consulting desks allowing easy consultation between the consultant(s) and junior doctors but seriously infringing patients' privacy. In the area around, there were rooms for simple biochemical tests, eye examinations, a secretary and a social worker. The medical team was supported by a senior sister and staff nurse, who spent time on non-clinic days giving dietary and other advice to new patients. Children attended on a separate day to spare them the distress of seeing the complications that might await them in adulthood. The first clinic exclusively for children was formally opened in 1936 by the Member of Parliament for Camberwell, Major Oscar Guest (1888–1958).[30]

Research

When Lawrence was appointed as a biochemist after Harrison left, the Committee of Management resolved that he be paid £375 per annum as from 1 April and that an honorarium of 10 guineas be paid in respect of the preceding two months (for comparison, the store boy in the engineering department was paid £32 10s per annum and the assistant in the Pathology Department £52 per annum). At this time, teaching hospitals typically had four full-time physicians who were elected by the governors. Being a gentleman and having uncontroversial political views were *sine qua non*s for election. Membership of the hospital Masonic Lodge also helped, although Lawrence himself had no interest in this. Physicians were not paid, but treated the sick poor and taught students. They made their money from private practice among the wealthy and aristocratic to whom they were introduced by the governors. With few exceptions, most teaching hospital physicians were not interested in research, and it was for this reason that the 1918 Haldane Report recommended setting up academic medical units headed by a full-time professor. By 1924, there were three: at Bart's, St Thomas' and University College Hospital.

Lawrence applied to the MRC for his first research grant in June 1924, noting that he was resident physician to a diabetic home in Highgate, where he also lived. He noted that

> so far I have had only a few [private] cases there in six months, and it is my hope in applying for this personal grant to be able to reduce private practice to a minimum and to undertake detailed research on a few hospital patients. I guarantee that my private work will not interfere with my research work.

His application was assessed by Henry Dale, who wrote

As to his qualifications for really original research work, I find it more difficult to form an opinion. I am sure that he is keen and competent to do work under direction, but I am not so certain as to his power of initiating good work for himself, now that Harrison has migrated to Great Ormond Street. My feeling however, is that Lawrence would be a justifiable speculation, to the extent of the grant which he asks, namely £200 [nearly £8,000 today] for one year. The programme which he suggests is by no means an unreasonable one, and he might even come across something quite exciting in trying the effect of Insulin on hyperthyroidism. If he proved disappointing as a research worker, we could probably manage to get good value out of him in connection with the proposed clinical testing [of the strength of insulin]. Altogether I think he would be a more promising investment than most.

T. R. Elliott (1877–1961),the newly appointed Professor of Medicine at University College Hospital, wrote

My inclination is to grant the £200. King's deserves help as a school. Lawrence does not push his claims. I see from the Directory that he collected several gold medals at Aberdeen, of which he makes no mention. Perhaps you might ask Harrison for a confidential statement of Lawrence's powers for independent work. He was associated with Harrison in several papers. Harrison receives a grant from the MRC and he is wise enough to be entrusted with the responsibility of reporting to the MRC on a prospective worker.

Harrison wrote a supportive letter saying, inter alia, that Lawrence was 'very keen to make himself efficient in scientific medicine'. He got the grant and treated four women with overactive thyroids with insulin.[31] Up to 100 units a day of insulin were given and elaborate measurements made of pulse rate, metabolic rate, etc. Three gained weight, which to Lawrence suggested 'the use of insulin in the treatment of under-nutrition and emaciation in cases other than diabetes and hyperthyroidism. It is probable that insulin will acquire a much wider therapeutic field with the progress of time.' This prediction came true, with insulin being used for severe vomiting of pregnancy and to stimulate nutrition in pulmonary tuberculosis and 'in the insane refusing food'.[32] Several papers reported good results when it was applied locally to wounds and one of the first of many papers reporting its use in bedsores was published in 1930.[33]

In 1934 Lawrence contributed a chapter on 'Heredity in diabetes mellitus and renal glycosuria' to *The Chances of Morbid Inheritance*, a 449-page book edited by the secretary of the Eugenics Society, Carlos P. Blacker, at whose wedding Lawrence had been best man.[34] He began by distinguishing between true diabetes and renal glycosuria (confusingly named diabetes innocens by George Graham). The latter was a symptomless inherited lowering of the renal threshold that was only important because it could be confused with diabetes if the blood sugar was not measured. It was usually discovered during life insurance examinations and had convincingly been shown to be inherited in a Mendelian dominant fashion.

Virtually every writer on diabetes in the late nineteenth and early twentieth centuries found a high frequency of positive family histories in their patients, and Lawrence thought that about 25% of cases were inherited. Strong evidence for a hereditary basis was the high concordance in homologous (identical) twins, with 7 of 11 in one series developing diabetes in the same year. Lawrence did not mention any examples known to him, but his successor at King's, David Pyke (1921–2001), collected a large series of diabetic twins in the 1960s and 70s.

Following the rediscovery of Mendel's work by the Cambridge zoologist William Bateson (1861–1926) in 1906, attempts were made to find human conditions that were inherited as dominants or recessives. Frustratingly, those which were found, such as alkaptonuria, cystinuria and brachydactyly, were very rare. In the 1920s and 30s, many diabetic specialists collected large families with diabetes and tried to fit them into recessive, dominant or X-linked recessive patterns. Lawrence had collected 54 families, which he submitted to a geneticist, Ruggles Gates (1882–1962), whom he knew through the Eugenics Society. Gates thought 5 were compatible with dominant inheritance and 19 with recessive (although a few were not entirely clear), and regarded the remaining 30 as irregular and conforming to neither type of inheritance. All 54 were also scrutinized by Lancelot Hogben (1895–1975), then Professor of Social Biology at the London School of Economics, who thought all were compatible with diabetes being produced by two dominant genes, situated in different chromosomes, both of which genes must be present to produce the disease. 'This', wrote Lawrence, 'may prove a fruitful hypothesis.'

Lawrence continued to be interested in the hereditary basis of diabetes, and in 1946 invited the geneticist Harry Harris (1919–94) to analyse the family histories of 1241 patients attending the juvenile and adult diabetic clinics at King's.[35] Harris concluded that older-onset cases were heterozygous for 'the gene' and young-onset cases homozygous for the same gene. He added for good measure the suggestion of incomplete penetrance depending on environmental factors and genetic background.

In his 1934 chapter, Lawrence pointed out that environmental factors were one of the ingredients that led 30 years later to diabetes being called the geneticist's nightmare. He wrote that

Another difficulty [in unravelling the genetics] is the undoubted influence of environment in the development of the disease. Over-eating and obesity, worry and mental overstrain may produce a disease which otherwise might have remained latent. As an example, the effect of under nutrition was clearly seen in all countries which suffered from a lack of food in the Great War, when the incidence of diabetes became definitely less, to rise again later. Hence the same hereditary defect in the islet tissue might or might not produce clinical diabetes according to the environment.

Lawrence did not himself have a family history of diabetes; none of his ancestors had suffered from the disease and there have been no cases yet in any of his 29 direct descendants at the time of writing.

References

1. Major RH. The treatment of diabetes mellitus with insulin. *J Am Med Assoc* 1923; **80**: 1597–600.
2. Maclean H. The use of insulin in general practice. *Lancet* 1923; **ii**: 829–33.
3. Lawrence RD. Local insulin reactions. *Lancet* 1925; **i**: 1125–6.
4. Lawrence RD. The effect of the prolonged use of insulin on the subcutaneous tissues. *Lancet* 1928; **i**: 1328.
5. Harrison GA, Lawrence RD, Marks HP. The strength of insulin preparations: a comparison between laboratory and clinical measurements. *Br Med J* 1925; **ii**: 1102–7.
6. Banting FG. Nobel Lecture 1923. In: *Nobel Lectures in Physiology or Medicine 1922–1941*. Amsterdam: Elsevier, 1965: 68.
7. Lawrence RD. Insulin therapy: successes and problems. *Lancet* 1949; **ii**: 401–5.
8. Harrison GA. Can insulin produce even a partial cure in human diabetes mellitus. *Q J Med* 1925–1926; **19**: 223–34.
9. Price FW. *A Textbook of the Practice of Medicine,* 2nd edn. Oxford: Oxford Medical Publications, 1926: 403–9. *Taylor's Practice of Medicine,* 13th edn. London: J & A Churchill, 1925: 571–6.
10. Lawrence RD. *The Diabetic Life: Its Control by Diet and Insulin.* London: J & A Churchill, 1925.
11. Editorial. Biochemistry and Medicine. *Lancet* 1923; **ii**: 791–2.
12. Oxley WHF. Blood sugar estimations by general practitioners. *Br Med J* 1923; **i**: 1115–16.
13. See Reference 10: 57–8.
14. Lawrence RD. A diabetic diet: the line ration scheme. *Br Med J* 1925; **i**: 261–2.
15. McCarrison R. A good diet and a bad one: an experimental contrast. *BMJ* 1926: **2**; 730–2.
16. Lawrence RD. Good and bad diets. *Br Med J* 1926; **ii**: 85.
17. Hugh Maclean (1883–1957). Chemical pathologist and later Professor of Medicine at St Thomas' Hospital.
18. Karl Petrén (1868–1927). Swedish physician and proponent of high-fat diets.
19. Section of Medicine. Results of insulin therapy in diabetes mellitus. *Br Med J* 1927; **ii**: 162–3.
20. Geyelin HR. Recent studies on diabetes in children. *Atlantic Med J* 1926; **29**: 825–30.
21. Sansum WD, Blatherwick NR, Bowden R. The use of high carbohydrate diets in the treatment of diabetes mellitus. *J Am Med Assoc* 1926; **86**: 178–81.
22. Rabinowitch IM. Experiences with a high carbohydrate–low calorie diet for the treatment of diabetes mellitus. *Can Med Assoc J* 1930; **23**: 489–98.
23. Lawrence RD. Diabetes: with special reference to high carbohydrate diets. *Br Med J* 1933; **ii**: 517–21
24. Fletcher AA, Campbell WR. The blood sugar following insulin administration and the symptom complex – hypoglycemia. *J Metab Res* 1922; **2**: 637–49.
25. Lawrence RD. Effect of exercise on insulin action. *Br Med J* 1926; **i**: 648-650.
26. Banting FG. Discussion on diabetes and insulin. *Br Med J* 1923; **ii**: 446.
27. Report of Meeting of Brighton and Sussex Medico-Chirurgical Society. *Br Med J* 1923; **ii**: 765.
28. Annotation. Edinburgh: Special outpatient clinics. *Lancet* 1924; **i**: 460–1.
29. Wauchope GM. *The Story of a Woman Physician*. Bristol: John Wright, 1963.
30. Medical News. *Br Med J* 1936; **ii**: 571.
31. Lawrence RD. Four cases of exophthalmic goitre treated with insulin: a preliminary report to the Medical Research Council. *Br Med J* 1924: **ii**: 753–5.

32. Short JJ. Increasing weight with insulin. *J Lab Clin Med* 1929; **14**: 330–5.
33. Joseph B. Insulin for bedsores. *Ann Surg* 1930; **92**: 318–19.
34. Blacker CP, ed. *The Chances of Morbid Inheritance*. London: HK Lewis, 1934.
35. Harris H. The familial distribution of diabetes mellitus: a study of the relatives of 1241 propositi. *Ann Eugen (Lond)* 1950; **15**: 95–110.

CHAPTER 6

Marriage and Family

I might so easily have gone through life without finding you

Lawrence to Anna Batson, 1927

In a letter home from India Lawrence had written that 'there are lots of pretty and lively girls here, but nothing fascinating to me. They are ephemeral and if they have any brains don't use them; and I have hardly met any interested in the arts, things that are best in life for me.' At the end of the war in 1918, he wrote to his parents saying that he had no thoughts of marriage. He wanted to get home and establish himself and become self-sufficient. Nine years later, in the spring of 1927, he met an intelligent and graceful young woman called Doreen Nancy Batson at a party in the village of Cotterstock in Northamptonshire. Her mother's pet name for her was Pearl but in adult life she became known as Anna as she disliked her given names.

Anna was born in Lancashire in 1902 where her father Thomas Batson (1852–1935), was Deputy Headmaster at Rossall School. He was a tall, strong sportsman who was selected to row for Oxford in the 1869 boat race but was forbidden from participating by his father who thought his son had a weak heart – a heart which actually lasted for 83 years. Anna's mother Elizabeth Christina Stretton (1876–1962) was born in Blennerville, County Kerry, daughter of a Harbour Master from Cork in southern Ireland. She trained as a nurse at Liverpool Royal Infirmary before working at Birkenhead Borough Hospital. Elizabeth was 24 years her husband's junior, but it was a long and happy marriage. Not long after their second child was born in 1905, Thomas Batson retired and the family moved to a large, comfortable house in Devon

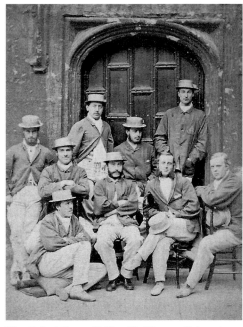

The Oxford Crew, 1869, with Thomas Batson top right.

surrounded by a large garden with numerous outhouses.

Anna was a warm, sociable girl who, according to her mother, could bear no confrontations but who loved animals, dancing, eurhythmics and all the performing arts. Many photographs in the family album show her in a dance pose or dressed in costume for a play. She was a pianist whose ambition to be a ballet dancer was thwarted by her height; she was 5 ft 9 in. Later, she studied Dalcroze eurhythmics and in 1921 spent some time at Liverpool College Huyton[1] before studying piano and violin at the Royal School of Music. She had an intelligent appreciation of poetry. During her teenage years she lovingly copied out many verses into a Commonplace book which included a quote from The Young Enchanted by Hugh Walpole: 'for true love the lust of the flesh must be added to the lust of the mind and the heart'.

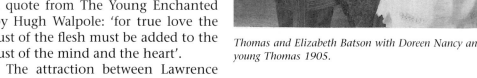

Thomas and Elizabeth Batson with Doreen Nancy and young Thomas 1905.

The attraction between Lawrence and Anna was instant and they wrote frequently during their enforced absences. Lawrence's letters are full of poetry and suffused with romantic imagery although in his very first letter he was hesitant and took a while to find his voice:

> *What a fine memory I have. I have remembered your address, your face and smile, caresses and scent, so now can set about writing to you.*

Not wanting to appear too eager he went on:

> *I haven't been thinking about you all the time, just occasionally you know and can't live perpetually in an atmosphere of love and romance. Can you?*

Early in their correspondence he assured her that:

> *I have you very tightly tied round my heart strings now.*

They both had a deep appreciation of nature and his letters are full of references to the moon and to sunsets, rippling water and quiet walks in countryside where he wishes she were by his side. He talks of a pale blue summer sky with silver

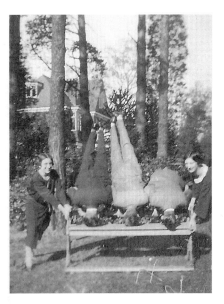

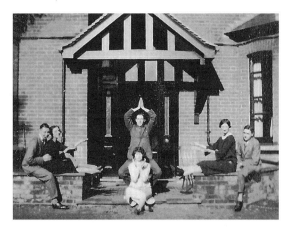

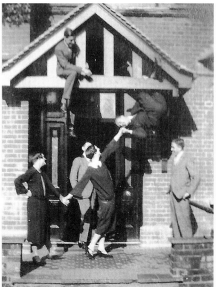

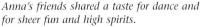
*Anna's friends shared a taste for dance and
for sheer fun and high spirits.*

ribbons or of a low dazzling sun in winter.
Later, gazing out of his window he asks if
she's seen the sunset 'glowing and really
beautiful' and longs for it to be reflected in
her face. When without her he describes
himself as 'sweetly sad and lonely' and asks
what has she done to him? He mentions
hard frost and fog outside 'but never within
me.' He told her that she epitomized his 'sense of romance, mystery and beauty'
going on to say that they 'must cultivate these together and grow a gorgeous rose
there from.'

Just over a year after Anna met Lawrence, he proposed to her on the banks of the
Serpentine on June 1st 1928 and later that night wrote:

> *Dearling, there is a silly business phrase 'to confirm our conversation of today' and
> I have just looked out and over the garden at our moon which blessed us at the
> Serpentine and want to say how happy I am and how fortunate in (having) you.
> What a full joyous and good life we shall lead.*

Her letter in return which began, 'you and me we are now and always each
other's beloved' went on to assure him that 'this tender love will be with us always.'
Her letter ended:

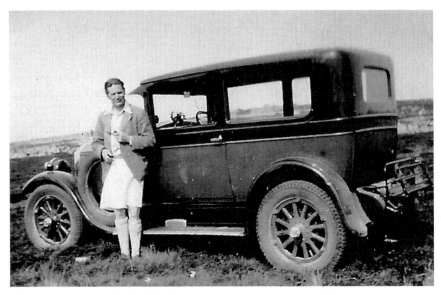

Lawrence in his courting days, 1928.

Robin love, you have come to mean so much to me and already you have brought such sweetness and beauty as I never hoped to find, our life together is going to be so fine and full.

Lawrence asked Thomas Batson for his daughter's hand in marriage. By 1928 it was known that diabetes ran in families but as Lawrence was the leading diabetes expert in the country any fears that Thomas might have had were allayed.

Of far more importance was that they shared many interests. They were an energetic pair who enjoyed tennis, the countryside, travel, dancing and both had a passionate love of music. Lawrence's taste was for classical but Anna's was broader and later she also came to love jazz and blues. The opening bars of Beethoven's 8th Symphony became a signal of mutual recognition, while the 7th Variation of Brahms' Variation on a theme of Haydn was a leitmotif that recurred through their lives together.

The wedding took place at Holy Trinity Church, Brompton followed by a reception in South Kensington. The best man was Victor Negus (1887–1974), the junior ENT surgeon from King's, who had won many medals and prizes. He contributed greatly to the advancement of surgery of the nose and throat and had been an usher at Lord Lister's funeral. Lawrence and Negus were vigorous sparring partners on both the tennis court and the billiard table and remained friends throughout their lives. Charles and Margaret Best attended the wedding. Best had come from Canada to study at the National Institute for Medical Research (NIMR) in London and the two couples became close friends

Lawrence would have preferred a simple registry office ceremony but Anna's upbringing had been a traditional Christian one so he agreed, reluctantly, to a

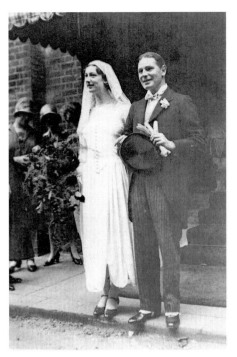

*Lawrence and Anna on their wedding day,
7 September 1928.*

church wedding. Church attendance had been a regular feature of his childhood in Aberdeen and his father was a Church elder but he had lost faith when so many of his friends were killed in the First World War.

When the couple returned from a seaside honeymoon, they lived in a small one bedroom flat in the KCH Student hostel at 143 Denmark Hill. Once married, there was no pressing economic need for Anna to work but she loved the interest and stimulus of being a repetiteur at the Rambert School of Ballet in Notting Hill Gate. Over the years she developed a close relationship with Madame Rambert and her debonair husband Ashley and also offered much support and help to the brilliant choreographer Antony Tudor (1908–1987) and his lifelong partner, the dancer Hugh Laing (1911–1988).

Lawrence and Anna spent their first married Christmas in Bordighera, a small

town on the Italian Riviera. It must have been quite a shock to return to London in that bitterly cold winter. Anna often mentioned that she felt she must have been a South Sea Islander in a previous life as she loved dancing, the sun, warm seas and eating fish and fruit. In February 1929 she wrote to congratulate the Bests on Charley's appointment as professor and head of department of Physiology at the University of Toronto in succession to JJR Macleod. Anna mentioned the recent Christmas holiday she'd had with her husband when:

> *The sun and flowers out there were lovely, and we played tennis and basked in the heat. Now of course we are in our winter Arctic[2], as you must be too. I expect you skate very well –*

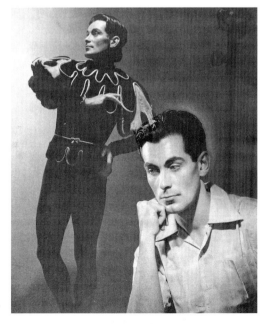

Signed 'To Anna, who gave me the push that started me off – with so many thanks and love, Hugh.

Robin is quite expert but I am very unversed in the art. It seems to require such an awful amount of practice to be any good. We have a dear small flat just near the hospital – only a few rooms but they are a good size and we look on to a garden which contains a singing robin sometimes.

1929 was a busy and productive year for both Lawrence and Anna. While working on his *Diabetic ABC* and *The Diabetic Life*, it was essential for him to know the precise composition of foods. His two-year collaboration at King's with the biochemist Robert McCance resulted in the publication of *The Carbohydrate Content of Food* which came to be regarded as a definitive text for many years. Lawrence's handbook The Diabetic ABC was published in 1929 and then on 1 June, at a nursing home in Maida Vale, their son Robert Thomas Batson Lawrence was born.

After a difficult birth, their joy in having a fine healthy boy can be imagined. Lawrence was 37 and became a loving and very active father who was, according to his middle son Adam, fascinated by his children, never ceasing to watch and to marvel at their development. As a severe

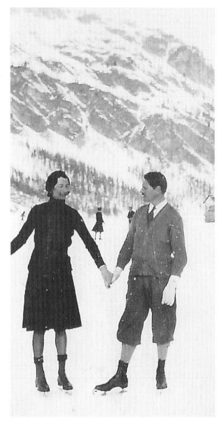

Lawrence and Anna at Sils in 1934.

diabetic he felt blessed to have children, let alone healthy ones. Soon after Rob's birth, he wrote to Charley Best:

My dear Best, yesterday we took the liberty of making you one of the godfathers to our son Robert Thomas Batson Lawrence – purely an honorary position and an attempt to express the part your work has played in my continuing existence. For family and other reasons we are not coming across this year but probably the BMA will see us next year in Canada.

After the baby's birth the Denmark Hill flat was too small because the Lawrences had employed a nanny trained under the strict regimen of Truby King, which promoted regular feeds, sleeps and bowel movements and discouraged cuddling the baby or giving him unnecessary attention. Rob and nanny went to live with Anna's parents near Battersea Park. Anna would spend the day with them before returning to the flat to be with Lawrence in the evening. This convenient arrangement, which gave the new parents uninterrupted nights, continued for a year until, in 1930, Lawrence bought a large family house at 63 Albert Bridge

Road in Battersea and the family were re-united. The location suited him well for driving to both King's and to Harley Street.

A typical working day in the 1930s started early. In the morning he did a long clinic followed by a ward round, as he had a few beds under his care. In the afternoon he would visit private patients in the London Clinic and see others in his consulting rooms in Harley Street. He might spend time in the lab at the London Clinic or visit a medical library. His books needed frequent revision and he would spend hours at his desk working on them. His first London club was the RAC but later he joined the Savile Club and was fond of dropping in there in the early evening to play snooker in the basement or enjoy stimulating conversations with friends such as H. G. Wells, Professor C. E. M. Joad, C. P. Snow and Huw Wheldon, who became Head of Documentaries and then Controller at the BBC. Lawrence could hardly have been in better company for the scientific and philosophical conversations he enjoyed so much.

By this time, Lawrence's private practice was flourishing and he was able to employ staff. There was a cook, butler, housemaid, nurse, gardener and, later, a chauffeur. Annual garden parties for children with diabetes were held here during the 1930s. They held two annual Christmas parties throughout the 1930s. The first was musical and after dinner the guests would go through to the drawing room and sit on gilded chairs. The second was a dance party and often guests came in fancy dress.

When he got home from work Lawrence and Anna would often unwind by playing piano pieces for four hands. They always loved playing together: Beethoven, Mozart, Schubert and also Gilbert and Sullivan arrangements. Lawrence's oft repeated aim on weekday evenings was to have an early night, a phrase which has passed down through the family. At weekends, they enjoyed entertaining and would invite their friends to dinners, parties and musical evenings. Lawrence had a fine tenor voice and sang from his battered old copy of *The Scottish Students' Song Book*. He also sang Schubert lieder to Anna's accompaniment. If he played a solo, it might be a Beethoven sonata full of mistakes, but delivered with flair and great élan.

The longest serving member of their staff was to be Gwen Amoore, a nurse

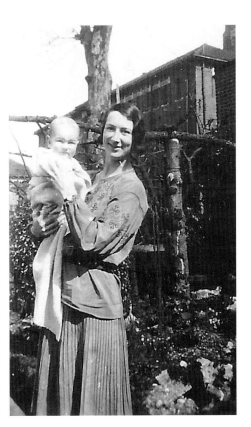

Anna and Rob in the garden of their flat by King's College Hospital.

at the Belgrave Children's Hospital, who joined as nanny in October 1932 when Anna was expecting her second child. Anna had not been happy with the rigidity of the Truby King system of baby and childcare and was much more comfortable with Gwen's firm but loving approach with her children. When the Lawrences went on holiday, Gwen would write a daily letter to them in the voice of the children, giving the smallest daily details that an absent parent appreciates hearing. She remained as the children's nanny until her marriage to Anna's brother Tim in 1940, but during the War the families lived next door to each other in a semidetached house in Wiltshire and Gwen continued to help with the boys there.

In July 1930, the distinguished writer and scientist H. G. Wells was referred to Lawrence by the controversial Dr Norman Haire (1892–1952), the first sexologist in

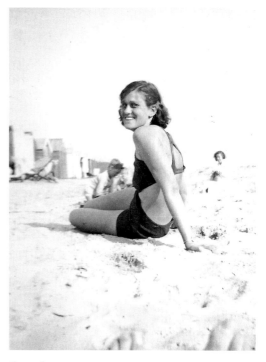

Gwen Amoore.

Harley Street. Haire was an Australian gynaecologist and birth control advocate who charged enormous fees for consultations. He came to England in 1919 and together with Countess Dora Russell, wife of the philosopher Bertrand Russell, organized the World League for Sexual Reform Congress at the Wigmore Hall where Wells was a delegate. Haire was self-aggrandizing and announced, 'Whatever my imperfections may be, I do not know of anybody else who has both the knowledge and the courage, to make him a better leader than myself in the movement for sexual reform'.

Lawrence had long admired Wells' work and wrote to his parents in 1918:

> *I finished your copy of Peter and Joan yesterday and enjoyed it very much. But Wells doesn't have much new to say for himself nowadays, but goes on repeating and amplifying his old ideas, which, of course, I always thought very sound and true. The only thing that struck me as really fresh was his analogy between the Ulster Anglicans and the German Junkers both of whom felt the race of life to be slipping past them and thought they must assert their creed and position by force of arms'.*

Recalling his first meeting, many years later, Lawrence noted that sugar had been found in Wells' urine. Two common symptoms of newly diagnosed diabetes in middle aged men are balanitis (irriation under the foreskin) and impotence.

Either would have been a major concern to a serial womaniser like Wells, who once explained to Charlie Chaplin:

There comes a moment in the day when you have written your pages in the morning, attended to your correspondence in the afternoon, and have nothing further to do. Then comes that hour when you are bored; that's the time for sex.

When Lawrence first examined Wells, he noted that H. G. was drowsy and unable to concentrate, which was not surprising considering how high his blood sugar was. However, since he did not have ketonuria, Lawrence thought 'he would slowly get rid of his sugar by diet restriction and loss of weight, which would also be good for his irregular heart (atrial fibrillation). Of course, I explained that I could clear the sugar temporarily at least by a few injections of insulin, but, after discussion, he said that he was going to be treated by diet alone in the first place although, as he said:

With my frequent habits of entertaining and being entertained, I shall often have to exert my will-power unpleasantly in restriction of appetites: this I am sure I can do and it will do my willpower good.' Wells must have taken his diabetes seriously because in three weeks he had lost 6lb, his urine was sugar free and his sexual problem had resolved.

In January 1931 Lawrence and Anna were invited to stay with Wells at his villa in the South of France. They accepted with 'pleasurable anticipation.' Before going, they received advice about life at the villa from Odette Keun, the Dutch writer who kept house for Wells, provided and enforced his diabetic diet, carried out his urine tests and 'provided more intimate personal requirements when mutually desired.' Odette's pet name for Wells was Pidou. Odette had written:

You will wonder what strangely dressed people you are going to meet. Pidou with his woolly Jaeger suiting and myself in my Arab donkey boy's burnous, but you will get accustomed to our unusual appearance. We never go out – I mean visiting – and unless you mean to visit Cannes, you need not bring smart clothes or an evening gown. But I must warn you that unlike the warm coast of the Riviera, up here at Grasse it is very cold in January and you must bring warm clothing. We have no central heating as Pidou dislikes it and blames it for clouding his brain, and our servants seem unable to keep the fires going or the windows tight shut.

Lawrence and Anna arrived at Cannes on the Blue Train. Lawrence wrote that:

It was certainly warm enough to line the coast with mimosa in full bloom. Odette was not in her Arab donkey-boy burnous but in smart French suiting which would have disguised her had we not known her in London. She was accompanied, not by H. G., but by his son, Anthony West, in a smart lounge suit. He took charge of our suitcases and, I'm glad to say, also the driving of the car. The guest villa was still warm as Charlie Chaplin and his wife had just left. After lunch at the villa, we

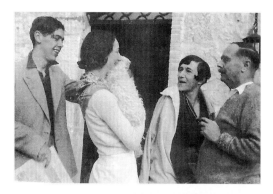

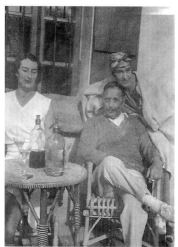

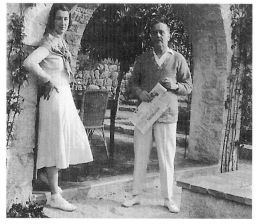

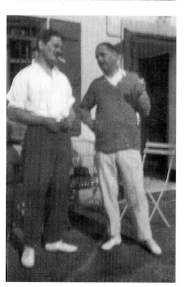

Photos from the Lawrence family album of the visit to HG Wells in the south of France.

realized that Odette's description of cold was correct, and we ran down to the guest house again to change into the warm clothing we had been warned to bring, and to keep the wood-fire going.

No records exist about Lawrence's treatment of Wells, and his diabetes is passed over very lightly in official biographies; indeed there is no mention of Lawrence in any of them, except in *H. G. Wells in Love*, the third volume of Wells' *Experiment in Autobiography* written in 1933. We know from Lawrence's notes that the two remained in close contact, especially towards the end of Wells' life.

Back in England, young Rob was being cared for by his maternal grandparents and a nanny. Adam Gay Lawrence was born at home on 20th May 1933 and Dan arrived three years later on 21st April 1936. The proud father clearly needed some rest and recuperation after the birth of his third son. He left Gwen Amoore and his mother-in-law with Anna, and went up to Aberdeenshire for a few days of fishing from where he wrote that he wishes he'd seen 'the first bathing of Dan' and enclosed a pressed primrose from the banks of the Dee. He thanked Anna for the remarks about 'the wonderful Father, but what about the loveliest and most perfect mother and lover – wife. I say so,' and he sent her 'a kiss, a birdsong, a sunlit hill, a primrose and endless love – but not a salmon.'

In their personal lives, it was a decade of arrivals and departures for the family. Between 1929 and 1936 there were three births and three deaths. Lawrence's exceptionally close relationship with his mother continued to the end of her life. On his 35th birthday she wrote:

It's a funny thing when your birthday comes round. I don't see you as grown up, you go back to being my darling baby boy for the time and I just love to think (and I can feel) you in my arms again.

Her pride and love shines through these last letters she wrote to him:

You have been, and are, to us all that a son could be and you've no idea how much your loving thoughtfulness for us has done to make these later years joyful.

Maggie Lawrence's asthma was always troublesome and she died in September 1932 aged 73, while staying with Lawrence's brother George in Worcestershire. Thomas returned to his native Aberdeen and died three years later aged 82.

Anna's father died aged 86 in 1933. She kept his last message to her written on her birthday in 1932 addressed to, 'My dearest most beloved girl.' The note went on to say that she had been their great blessing and had only ever given them joy and ended, 'God bless you from your old Dad.' The stereotype of the distant, authoritarian Victorian patriarchs was certainly not true in either Lawrence's or Anna's case.

The Lawrence's GP, Dr Leonard Haydon, delivered both younger boys and over the years the two families became close friends. In 1933 Lawrence and Anna visited Hayling Island in Hampshire with a view to taking a house there for the summer. It would be an easy journey for Lawrence's weekend visits and they rented a house for 12 weeks. It was a glorious summer and they were delighted with life there. They looked for a house to buy but instead bought a plot of land with the Haydons on the northern side of the island. Through their friends the architectual writer, journalist and businessman Geoffrey Boumphrey and his wife Esther, they had met the modernist New Zealand born architects Amyas Douglas Connell and his brother-in-law Basil Ward, who had been deeply influenced by the work of Le Corbusier. The two families commissioned them to build two adjoining houses and, as Basil Ward said later, 'You can imagine how exciting it was for two young architects full of Corbusier's ideas to get a commission like that.'[3] In 1933 Connell and Ward joined Colin Lucas to form the Connell, Ward & Lucas architectural practice which built around 20 private houses in England in the 1930s using a

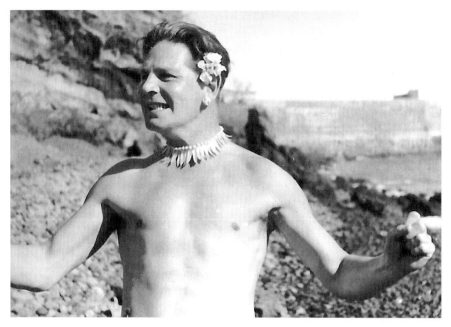

Lawrence on holiday. Close examination of the photograph reveals the criss-cross scars on Lawrence's abdomen from the series of operations he had between 1914 and 1916.

reinforced concrete construction. For Corbusier, a house was a 'machine for living' and these light, open, airy houses embodied the new ideas about healthy living. All clutter and general knick-knackery was swept away. The floors were unjointed using cork or linoleum. With the aim of clean lines and simplicity, the built-in furniture was neatly fitted using plywood. Surfaces were hard, smooth and easy to clean. There were sunroofs, terraces, large windows and garden doors. Everything was conducive to outdoor living. In the late 1920s, a suntan began to be seen as a glow of well-being from a healthy outdoor life, rather than the mark of the rural poor.

Planning permission was received in March 1934 and the houses were built during that summer. The Lawrences named theirs 'Saltings' and it was ready for occupation in the autumn. It was painted pale peach and was set a little further back from the Haydon's house, which created a large open space between the two. The south-facing front rooms had extensive glazing and were flooded with light. The rooms at the back had views over a small orchard down the long garden towards the foreshore and the expanse of Langstone Harbour and distant views across to Butser and Portsdown Hills and the western end of the South Downs. Geoffrey Boumphrey had co-founded Finmar, a company that imported Alvar Aalto's furniture from Finland.[4] It was the height of modernism and was made of natural and organic materials, mainly wood. The family would go down at weekends throughout the summer and spend the whole of August there. Friends would join them and a childhood memory of Adam's is of Hugh Laing the ballet

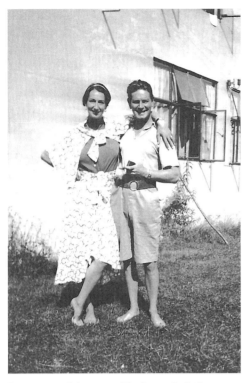

Lawrence and Anna outside the newly built 'Saltings' – the house that was to become such a special place for the family.

dancer doing arabesques on the bar of the children's swing and also on the parapet of the roof terrace which was 6 metres off the ground.

There was a hard tennis court in the garden. Lawrence and Anna were both keen players and as the boys grew up they played family foursomes. Later, Lawrence became keen on real tennis, as there was an old court on Hayling Island which was restored in the early 1950s and all the boys took this up enthusiastically. Both Adam and Dan played real tennis for the university when at Cambridge.

One of the great golfing attractions for the Haydon and Lawrence families was the classic links course on the Solent at Hayling. Lawrence, playing off a handicap of around 15, had a simple but effective style of running swing with a

high finishing flourish learned in his Aberdeen youth. He would toss the ubiquitous cigarette onto the edge of the tee, take his shot and then collect the smouldering stub and continue smoking it. He maintained that at one time or another he'd completed all the short holes on the Hayling course in one. Anna wasn't a keen golfer but enjoyed walking round the course with him. All three boys were given lessons by the resident Scottish pro and Adam counts the family golf rounds on Hayling as some of the happiest times in his childhood. Lawrence loved the views over to the Isle of Wight and watching the skylarks and butterflies.

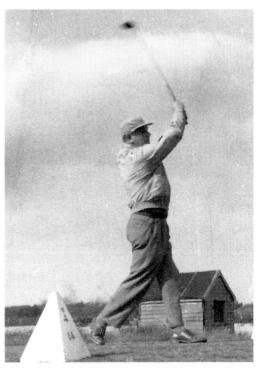

Lawrence on the links at Hayling Island.

Lawrence and Anna became keen filmmakers in the 1930s and their footage captures wonderful family holidays at 'Saltings'. It should be remembered that the movie camera only came out on bright sunny days and so it presents a charming concentration of outdoor family life. There are no clips of bored boys lounging inside and squabbling during the drizzle, but rather a stream of perfect summer activities is recorded. The brothers sailing model boats, pushing a rowing boat onto millpond-calm waters, diving, whirling around on an improvized swing with a barrel, lighting fires, making camps, riding pedal cars or bikes, doing acrobatics, pulling each other round on a small wagon, and playing with a train set. When they were older, there was a sailing dinghy. The boys loved sports: badminton, croquet, quoits, tennis, hockey and cricket all feature in the films, as well as much general larking around with sticks or play fights with their father or doing target practice with small rifles.

An incident that wasn't captured on film took place on Lake Como in the early 1950s when staying at the lakeside villa of their friends the Tomlinsons. Lawrence, a confident and versatile sportsman, rashly assumed greater sailing ability than he actually possessed. On a calm summer day, he took the teenage Adam sailing in a Flying 15 but when a sudden and violent storm blew up, Lawrence lost control. They capsized and very nearly drowned. Any restorative sugar was quickly washed away but they managed to cling to the upturned yacht for two hours before a passing ferry picked them up.

Lawrence and Anna shared progressive ideas about education. Lawrence himself had a highly traditional, competitive and rigorous education in Aberdeen at the Grammar School and then at the University. He complained bitterly about the outdated rigidity of some of the teaching on his university course where one professor simply read from his notes or from a book to the captive audience who had no escape as there was compulsory registration at the beginning of every

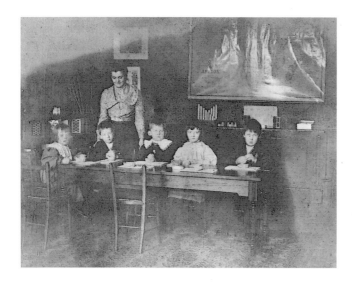

Anna in white smock. The children all have modelling clay and rolling pins and there is a map and other educational aids on the shelf behind.

lecture. Despite his private practice, domestic staff, smart car and comfortable lifestyle, Lawrence was a committed liberal and democrat, the product of the Scottish Enlightenment, and did not approve of traditional public schools. Anna had been brought up in a family with a strong public school tradition on her father's side, but had known much freedom in her rural childhood. From the photograph on page 114, it is probable that she was educated at home for the early part of her schooling.

Lawrence and Anna heard about a school called Beltane in Wimbledon, which was based on Montessorian principles and was part of the progressive movement in education. The Beltane School was founded by Andrew and Joan Tomlinson (known to everyone as the Tommies)[5] and opened in Wimbledon in May 1934. Andrew was an economist with no schoolteaching experience. His wife Joan had graduated with a first in psychology from Cambridge and had taught at a secondary boys' school in south London. They had worked with the WEA (Workers' Educational Association) in Yorkshire, teaching miners and factory workers at the end of their shift. The Tommies had been turned down for the joint headship at King Alfred's School, Hampstead, founded some 30 years earlier by a group of parents described by Joan as 'Fabians, artists and sandaled intellectuals', so the couple founded their own school where their four children could also attend. There was an anomaly, as the Tommies were socialists who had even backed the motion to abolish private schools.

The first pupils at Beltane were mostly from middle class families of intellectuals – doctors, journalists, writers and architects. Later, they took some troubled children from local authority schools who had been refused entry elsewhere.

The Tommies wanted to achieve the highest possible standards, both educational and material: 'if children studied music they must meet and learn from musicians of standing; in art they should find inspiration from real artists and craftsmen.' Edmund Rubbra (1901–1986), the distinguished British composer, was their first music teacher, and Arthur Wragg (1903–1976), the socialist, pacifist illustrator taught art at Beltane during the war when he was a conscientious objector.

Unlike one or two schools in the progressive movement, Mrs. Tommie noted that everyone at Beltane took it for granted that they went to lessons: 'it's what schools are for, to teach you.' Anna and Lawrence were attracted to a school that encouraged children to become reasonably polite and considerate while inculcating a respect for scholarship and an interest in the political affairs of the school. With the relatively mixed intake of pupils, the Tommies believed it was especially important that children should develop sympathy and tolerance for the frailties and eccentricities of others.

Ernie Weiss (1932–2006), an ex Beltane pupil, wrote a thoughtful appraisal of his time there, which summed up its ethos. He wrote that:

a key aim in Beltane was to offer children a happy environment and to present learning as a pleasurable and positive experience. The Tommies also set out to promote the pupil's innate curiosity, imagination and creativity. These are a child's most valuable assets, which conventional schooling is more likely to stifle.

Weiss went on to say:

> *While the Tommies were sympathetic to the philosophy of child-centred development, unlike some progressives, they also had a high regard for scholarship and academic excellence… The Tommies fostered mutual respect for both people and property and promoted social skills, with decent, considerate and courteous behaviour as the norm.*

The Tommies had a strong commitment to the creative and performing arts. They also were keen and knowledgeable art historians who passed their passion on to many of their pupils.

It was also during this period that Lawrence set off on his first international venture. On September 7th 1936 he and his neighbour Dr. Leonard Haydon left Hayling Island for Southampton and boarded the Canadian Pacific steamship liner *Empress of Australia* en route for Canada.

He was delighted to meet some of the actors who were travelling to New York to perform in Hamlet on Broadway with Leslie Philips. His new friends were the King, Polonius, Laertes and the Gravedigger. Ophelia (Pamela Stanley) was 'bright and pretty enough.'

Charley Best met them in Toronto and took them to the guest quarters at Hart House, a residential college hall. 'There are no students about yet, so we have the place, swimming pools all to ourselves.' Best, a keen rider since boyhood, kept horses on a neighbouring farm. 'Horses used for diphtheria and other sera and used for riding too!' Lawrence, the keen and competent rider from the Indian days 'felt a little nervous' when he and Best set off on horseback but quickly regained his confidence.

Best then took him to his 'beautiful research place and I saw the old benches where Banting and he discovered insulin. I found myself rather touched, as at a shrine, for the first time in any laboratory.' The lovely day continued with a game of golf and a 'marvellous pinky sunset and

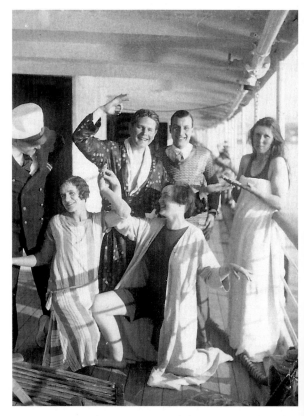

Lawrence joining the actors on board the Empress of Australia.

newish moon.' At Best's labs he saw 'all sorts of interesting things' but we don't hear what they were. He reported that 'I have now met most of the Toronto insulin people, a fine lot, and there is an important new development in protamine insulin which it was worth coming to see.' He presumably had met David Scott (1892–1971) and Albert Fisher at the Connaught Laboratories, who had developed protamine zinc insulin. He said he was sorry to leave Toronto, 'where we had a v happy time among honest, intelligent and jolly people. Best and Banting have a fine lot of keen young workers and enough money for full equipment, the profits from American insulin, though they personally draw not a penny.'

Lawrence and Leonard Haydn then travelled to Boston in style on the train in 'a "drawing room" sleeper which we had to ourselves.' He noted that 'the country behind Boston looked like England, mildly hilly and wooded'. He was not impressed with the clam broth that was offered at breakfast, 'a revolting drink of salt and sordidness – one sip enough.'

Joslin had arranged accommodation for them at 'a very dignified old University Club (the Harvard Club of Boston) and he ended his letter with 'tomorrow the great Joslin's clinic at last.' Lawrence described Joslin as 'a brisk, alert, thin man of 67 who rushed us about at high speed in his fine hospital. But I learned nothing and was frankly disappointed at first meeting.' They were shown around Boston and Harvard in brilliant sunshine. That evening, he was to attend a dinner at Joslin's house 'to meet his group and a few other pundits. They expect me to talk I believe and I hope to get something out of them.' He didn't seem too hopeful though, adding, 'at any rate we shall go on to New York tomorrow night and I am sure that city will be a thrill.'

New York inspired him. He lunched with a 'Dr [Elaine] Ralli, female, who then took us to her hospital.' He met an English Professor of Medicine at the Arbury Club, walking up the flashing advertisements of Broadway, and wrote later, 'Just back from a marvellous outing with an English biochemist, on the top of the Rockefeller Building, 85 storeys up.' They went to the observation roof 'in a three quarter moon and all sparkling New York and the neighbouring islands brillianted (*sic*) with lights and rivers and waterways showing them up. Many of the highest buildings, one a thousand feet, are spoiled by decorative towers on top, but others are simple and beautiful and the whole aspect most thrilling. It was difficult to get me back here by midnight.' He told Anna that New York was full of 'beauty parlors but not a single beauty like you, my Annabel.'

The next day he was in Baltimore staying quietly two miles from the city with E. Cowles Andrus (1896–1978),[6] a Cardiologist at the Johns Hopkins Hospital who had worked with Henry Dale in London in the 1920s. He was glad to have such cosy respite after the whirl of New York and was hoping to get Mrs. Andrus to play two handed piano pieces with him, 'there are plenty of *our* duets about, which belonged to her mother.' He was thrilled to have purchased a Packard car in America and hired a driver to take him to Baltimore. He described the car in loving detail telling her it would 'take us up and down to Hayling in grand fashion.' His plan was to have it loaded onto the ship on their homeward crossing.

Once again, he was unimpressed by the hospital where he 'saw the diabetic man, very poor show I thought, but some other interesting men.' He recorded a quiet evening, 'a lot of talk, some bridge and Andrus singing folk songs of all countries to his lute'.

In Rochester, Minnesota, Lawrence spent three days at the Mayo Clinic. He found Rochester to be the 'greatest contrast to the rushing roaring cities I have been in lately and you have to go only half a mile in any direction to be in a peaceful undulating country where agriculture is decorated by copses of these trees and scarlet dogwood.' Next, he was to be very impressed by his visit to the Mayo, 'this is the greatest medical centre I have yet been in and fairly humming with patients and the brightest brained doctors I have ever met. The whole town is a hospital and I suppose 90% of the people in this hotel are patients or their relatives.' He was fascinated to discover there was a dietetic restaurant 'where you can walk in and eat your diet correctly'. This had been inaugurated by Dr Will Mayo in the early 1920s, the rationale being that 'patients learned better with their eyes than their ears.' One day there Lawrence described as follows:

Breakfast at 7.30 a.m. in diet restaurant with Dr. [Russell] Wilder [1885–1959] the chief man on my subject and metabolism here; then to one hospital (there are three) where the day started at 8 a.m. with a 'seminar', a meeting of the staff and graduate students to demonstrate and discuss the pet cases of the week. Very keen and interesting and I was asked to talk and let them have it hot and strong for 20 minutes. Then to two other hospitals to see cases. Then to the diabetic outpatients until nearly 1 pm. Lunch party of chief people interested in diabetes in the diet restaurant.

All this was followed by discussions and a cocktail party and reception in a surgeon's house and a dinner 'de luxe' at the hotel. Lawrence was clearly impressed by Russell Wilder who, 'looked after us like a father, brother, aide de camp and valet all combined – a great fellow.'

His trip finished with a visit to St Paul for the 21st Annual International Assembly of the Inter-State Post graduate Medical Association of

English Surgeon Offers New Diabetes Diagnosis – would take blood from ear lobe instead of Arm.

The report went on, 'An eminent English surgeon, himself afflicted with the disease, today advanced a new method for diagnosing diabetes before 1200 delegates to the international medical assembly. Dr Robert D Lawrence of King's College Hospital in London suggested the blood used in examinations be taken from the ear lobe instead of from a vein in the arm. "This is like catching a sugar train before it reaches a town instead of catching the train after it returns from the town where the sugar has been unloaded," he said. He believed such a practice would greatly reduce the percentage of doubtful cases. In making the test the patients are given a large dose of sugar. The blood is examined every half hour for two hours. The results are compared to the reactions of normal persons and thus the extent of the disease can be more accurately determined. Diabetes was increasing, Dr. Lawrence held, because of "a greater abundance of food in the world. Most of us are better fed than we were twenty years ago", he said, "Obesity induces diabetes and we appear to be eating more than is good for us."'

North America.[7] Lawrence was one of 90 speakers and his photo was included in the paper under the caption 'Famed Doctors Greeted.' (See insert of press report) After this he returned to New York and boarded the ship bound for Southampton.

Evidently the Packard couldn't be unloaded and put through customs in time for him to drive it away from the gangplank but it became the family car for many years.

The Lawrence's close and comfortable family life was soon to be disrupted with the declaration of war in September 1939.

References

1. Drawing certificate, 1919.
2. According to the BBC weather records, in Mid February 1929, a bitter easterly wind brought persistent frost. The temperature at Ross-on-Wye fell to – 17°C, (1°F). There were considerable stretches of the River Thames in London that were frozen over.
3. Quoted in Connell, Ward and Lucas: 'A Modernist Architecture in England' Dennis Sharp, Sally Rendel.
4. Davis K. Scandinavian Furniture in Britain: Finmar and the UK market 1949 – 1952. *J Design Hist* 1997; **10**: 39–52.
5. Ernie Weiss was educated at Beltane and has written a detailed and informative account of his time at the school.
6. E. Cowles ('Coke') Andrus was a worldwide leader in cardiology and was instrumental in its development as an independent medical discipline and major component of modern medicine. A faculty member at Johns Hopkins for more than 50 years, he made significant contributions to heart research, teaching, and patient care. Dr. Andrus was the first director of the Cardiology Division, served as Assistant Dean of the Medical Faculty, and founded and directed the Cardiovascular Division.
7. Press cutting from Lawrence's scrap book.

CHAPTER 7

New Insulins, New Challenges

In 1932, Lawrence was promoted to junior physician in charge of the Diabetic Department and was awarded the Fellowship of the Royal College of Physicians (FRCP). In 1935, a research fellowship was established in the Diabetic Clinic, funded by a donation from the Sir Halley Stewart Trust. In the same year, a gift of £500 was received on the condition that nine other similar sums were given, for the creation of a ward for diabetic patients. Such a ward was included in the hospital development programme and in 1936 Lawrence himself promised £3000 and the House Committee put £16000 into the programme. By 1938, an architect was instructed to proceed with drawings for the building of a ward combining public-funded and private patients, children and adults, to be built on the second floor above the Diabetic Clinic.

In April 1939, a tender of £9190 for the construction was accepted. In September of that year, the House Committee approved the continuation of the building, as it was near completion, 'so long as the builders were able to obtain supplies'. The onset of the Second World War resulted in £300 extra costs, and a further £800 was required for equipment. One item of equipment, which is so taken for granted today, was the purchase of a 'Frigidaire' for the diabetic kitchen – the House Committee approved the purchase on the condition that Lawrence raised the £55 necessary.

In November 1939, it was noted that the new diabetic ward should be opened as soon as possible, which was achieved on 29 June 1940. The accommodation consisted of 16 beds, including private ones, a cot, and a separate room for treating diabetic coma. In 1939, Lawrence was appointed physician-in-charge of the Diabetes Department, having served seven years as assistant physician – a standard procedure of the hospital.

By the beginning of the 1930s, many of the practical day-to-day problems of living with insulin had been resolved, apart from the need for two or three injections a day. What most patients and many doctors wanted was an insulin that could be given once a day and then forgotten. Attempts had been made in the 1920s to lengthen the action of insulin, but had failed because of poor stability, painful injections or variability of absorption. The problem was solved in 1936 by Hans Christian Hagedorn (1888–1971) in Copenhagen.[1] His aim was, by moving its isoelectric point, to develop an insulin that was relatively insoluble in tissue fluid. This was finally achieved by combining it with protamine from the sperm of the rainbow trout. The first preparation was not stable and, when marketed in 1936 as Insulin Leo Retard, was sold in packets of six ampoules, five of which contained protamine insulin and the sixth a phosphate buffer. The patient would prepare enough for a few days by injecting buffer into the vial containing the acid solution of protamine insulin.

Hagedorn gave supplies of his new insulin to Lawrence, who reported his results in 1936.[2] Hagedorn usually gave soluble insulin in the morning to cover meals and protamine insulin at night to control the fasting blood sugar. Lawrence thought some patients might find the use of two sorts of insulin confusing and aimed to find out if protamine insulin could be used as a once-daily insulin. After trials on a few patients, he agreed with Hagedorn that, although it lasted up to 24 hours and could control fasting blood sugar, it was not strong enough to control hyperglycaemia after meals. He thought what was needed was 'another insulin preparation combining the qualities of ordinary and protamine insulinate'. Another thing he noticed in his patients was that protamine insulin caused 'less symptoms of hypoglycaemia, even at the same blood sugar concentration'.

Following Hagedorn's success with protamine insulin, several more long-acting preparations were introduced in the next 20 years, starting with protamine zinc insulin (PZI), which was developed in 1936 by David Scott (1892–1971) and Albert Fisher in Charles Best's section of the Connaught Laboratories; they found that a surplus of protamine and a small amount of zinc could stabilize the neutral protamine insulin.[3] This preparation lasted up to 72 hours, but if given alone its action did not begin for 9 or 10 hours and was not strong enough to overcome hyperglycaemia after breakfast the next morning. This could be overcome by adding soluble insulin, but, if they were mixed in the same syringe, the results were unpredictable because the excess zinc converted some of the soluble insulin into PZI. To many clinicians, the great advantage of PZI was that many, or even most, patients could now be treated with one injection a day. Lawrence described it as the *practitioner's insulin* for choice' [italics in original].[4] His article extolled the simplicity of the new method; for a newly diagnosed patient, he suggested that the first step was to find what he called 'the *basal* dose, that which will continue its action for twenty four hours and keep the blood sugar *normal before breakfast* and yet cause no hypoglycaemia during the night'. For mild cases, a single dose was often enough, but for more severe cases, soluble insulin had to be added. He noted, as many patients and physicians soon discovered, that hypoglycaemic symptoms were 'slower in onset and less obvious to the patient'. With time, it became apparent that PZI could cause severe warningless hypoglycaemia, especially at night.

Russell Wilder (1885–1959) of the Mayo Clinic had personal experience of the problem of warningless hypoglycaemia on long-acting insulins. In 1936, he went to the Annual Convention of the American Medical Association in Kansas City with his assistant Dr Randall Sprague (1906–90) and a dietician, Miss Nelson, both of whom had diabetes. On the second evening, Dr Sprague could not be found and Wilder eventually located him wandering in the streets distractedly, 'in a delayed reaction from protamine insulin'. On the drive home, they stopped at a hotel, where Miss Nelson was unable to write her name in the register because of hypoglycaemia. It took some persuasion to convince the innkeeper that she was not drunk. This must have made quite an impression on Wilder, who later quoted one of his patients as saying, after going onto PZI, 'I don't have diabetes any more;

I have insulin reactions.' He went so far as to advise patients on PZI not to sleep alone.[5] Lawrence's comment about changing people to PZI was:

I do not make the change in the case of the hundreds of patients who have lived a healthy and contented life for months or years on two doses a day [of soluble insulin] which they find no great inconvenience. I also refuse to do so with some patients who are careless or lead very irregular lives: the continuous action of the depot insulin, unbalanced by the necessary frequent small meals, makes them more liable to hypoglycaemia than when two smaller doses of soluble insulin are taken before breakfast and the evening meal.

Even when their doctors were enthusiastic, many patients rejected the new insulins. One was the chest physician Charles Fletcher (1911–95), who developed diabetes in 1940 – an eventful year in which he also got married and gave the world's first penicillin injection! As he described it:[6]

At first I took long acting insulin (protamine zinc), but I found this socially intolerable. It demands an evening meal at a fixed time which is often impracticable, especially after going to a theatre or in foreign countries where dinner may be very late. Twice daily soluble insulin led to frequent late morning hypoglycaemia. At my wife's suggestion I started doing what the normal pancreas does and went over to three injections of soluble insulin daily before my main meals, supplementing the evening dose with a little isophane to cover the next early morning. I take extra insulin supplements to control unusual hyperglycaemia.

In 1963, Lawrence explained that:[7]

When the introduction of a long-action insulin made the treatment by one daily injection a possibility, many refused its trial, saying that they were quite happy and understood their treatment – as did their doctors – and its adjustment. If on admission to some hospital after an accident or minor operation they were transferred to a one-dose treatment by an enthusiastic junior hospital doctor who thought the latest must be the best, they mostly came to me in a few weeks asking to return to their previous treatment because they were showing sugar and having hypoglycaemia at puzzling times. And so they went on year after year with some 150 g of carbohydrate and minor adjustments of insulin – the commonest dose being some 20 units morning, 16 units evening – and a full life of work and vigorous play.

Irrespective of whether they were on PZI or unmodified soluble insulin, Lawrence noted in a 1941 paper that:[8]

as years of insulin life go on, sometimes only after 5 to 10 years, I find it almost the rule that the type of insulin reaction changes, the premonitory autonomic symptoms are missed out and the patient proceeds directly to the more serious manifestations involving the nervous system.

So, for example, if a meal was late, instead of sweating and shaking, the patient would become obstreperous, create a scene and refuse sugar. The same patient might sometimes have warning symptoms and at other times be completely unaware that his blood sugar was low. 'It is obvious', wrote Lawrence, 'that these are serious dangers'. He could not explain this change, but indicated ways in which patients might avoid hypoglycaemia in the first place: these included the suggestion that urine tests should never be continuously sugar-free throughout 24 hours, reflecting modern teaching on relaxation of blood glucose control. He was well aware of the dangers of hypoglycaemia and driving, advising the need for both careful education of the patient, and stressing the vital importance of carrying emergency carbohydrate in the vehicle when driving.[9]

Infrequently, hypoglycaemia can be fatal. Lawrence, with his perpetual scientific curiosity, examined at post mortem the brains of six patients who had died from hypoglycaemia, two of whom had been on insulin coma treatment for schizophrenia (one had been given 300 units of insulin on 22 occasions, leading to convulsions on 6 of them). Widespread degeneration and necrosis of nerve cells and other changes were described.[10]

In 1934, Lawrence was invited by the *Lancet* to contribute an article on the prognosis of diabetes in children.[11] The disease was no longer inevitably fatal. In fact, of 164 patients under 16 years of age treated since 1923 by Joslin's associate Priscilla White, 147 were still alive in 1928. Lawrence had treated 59 under-16s as hospital patients with 6 deaths, and 69 as private patients with only 1 death. He stressed that such results needed 'continuous care and a routine of controlled diet and insulin'. Uncontrolled children sometimes developed cataracts and large livers and 'some workers declare that most of these children develop arteriosclerosis, minor but appreciable by refined methods of examination'. He did not go into further detail, but what he was referring to is what are now called specific diabetic complications such as retinopathy. Retinopathy had been first described in the middle of the nineteenth century and the most comprehensive description was given by the famous German ophthalmologist Julius Hirschberg (1843–1925) in 1890. He wrote that 'In careful, repeated examination a few haemorrhages can be found in most diabetics with a duration of the diabetes from 6 to 10 years.'[12] The only people who survived diabetes for more than 6 years were middle-aged people who also had arteriosclerosis, and for the next 40 years it was assumed that hardening of the arteries caused retinopathy. This view gradually changed during the 1930s with a 1934 paper by Henry Wagener, Thomas Dry and Russell Wilder of the Mayo Clinic being particularly influential. They examined all the patients in their clinic and found a few, usually young, who had retinal haemorrhages but no other clinical evidence of vascular disease (i.e. calcification of vessels on X-rays). They concluded that:[13]

> *In the large majority of cases of diabetes, however, whether hypertension is present or not, lesions of the retina, if present, are characteristic of diabetes and are not seen in similar form or distribution in any other disease ... [furthermore] ... The very existence of retinitis in cases in which patients have no other signs of vascular*

disease must mean that diabetes alone does something to injure the finer arterioles or venules of the retina, probably the latter.

The problem of complications in young diabetics became increasingly obvious during the late 1930s and early 1940s. The sense of doom was articulated by the Canadian physician Israel Rabinowitch (1890–1983), who wrote in 1944:[14]

There is nothing more disturbing than the diabetic who acquires the disease in childhood; who apparently is a picture of robust health – who looks and feels perfectly well – but whose blood vessels have been degenerating insidiously for years; who, in the early 20s or 30s and probably married and with a family, is beginning to feel the effect of the degenerative changes, either because of a progressive hypertension, kidney failure, disturbance of sight due to retinitis or a sudden attack of coronary thrombosis.

Lawrence kept a book in which he made detailed drawings of his patients' eyes over the decades and also wrote several papers on diabetes and the eyes. Refractive changes in response to increases or decreases in blood sugar had been reported many times. In 1932, Lawrence was clearly irked by a wordy paper by an ophthalmic surgeon Reginald Affleck Greeves (1878–1966) about two middle-aged women who had been able to discard their glasses when they developed diabetes. Greeves thought that this was rare, but Lawrence wrote:[15]

I find such changes extremely common in patients who are rapidly de-sugared by diet and insulin, and have formed the impression that they occur in some degree and for a short time in nearly 50% of such diabetics over 45 years of age. In them reduction of the blood sugar to normal unmasks a presbyopia which the myopic effect of hyperglycaemia had compensated. Younger patients show these changes much more rarely.

He had seen this in 200 patients, and made it his practice to warn people that it might occur, 'otherwise,' he wrote, 'they are apt to think that insulin is making them blind'.

In 1936 with an ophthalmologist, Harold Levy (1875–1977), he described a patient aged 59 with poorly controlled diabetes who had vascularization of the iris (rubeosis iridis), apparently the first description of this rare complication of proliferative retinopathy.[16] In 1943, Lawrence was the principal speaker at a meeting at the Royal Eye Hospital, where, according to the report, 'he described the changes he had observed in many thousands of diabetic eyes.'[17] He estimated that 15% of his patients, mostly elderly, had retinopathy and 'in many it is already established when the diabetes is diagnosed'. He did not mention the tragedy of a young person becoming blind from proliferative retinopathy, so presumably he had not seen such a case at this point. He ended his talk by chiding ophthalmologists 'who do not test urines or measure blood pressures and I do not see how without doing this they can come to an accurate diagnosis, increase their knowledge and help the patients'. Some things never change! In 1948, he described two women with acute haemorrhagic retinopathy in pregnancy.[18] The first, who had been on insulin for 19 years, was 'a spirited and clever young woman who led the wildest of diabetic lives, travelling all over the world'. This was associated with poor control, so she was 'a perfect candidate for retinal and other complications which long-standing and especially uncontrolled diabetes often brings'. In both patients, the eye changes resolved completely within a year or two.

In 1949, Lawrence wrote that:[19]

> twenty years ago I taught the students that many elderly diabetics developed the triad of retinopathy, albuminuria (with or without hypertension) and gangrene, commonly all present together. And now to watch this same picture, though without gangrene, develop in more and more young patients is a tragedy and a challenge.

He asked rhetorically:

> Does clinical experience show that the worst controlled cases develop vascular complications earlier and more often than the better controlled?

The answer was almost certainly 'yes'.

He returned to the question in 1963 in an article entitled 'Treatment of 90 severe diabetics with soluble insulin for 20–40 years'.[20] He had been impressed by a study from Malmö, Sweden, in which Johnsson compared the frequency of complications in 56 patients diagnosed between 1922 and 1935 and in 104 diagnosed between 1935 and 1945.[21] Those diagnosed before 1935 had a strict diet and multiple daily injections of insulin and were told to aim for sugar-free urine. Those diagnosed after 1935 were on a free diet and glycosuria was ignored provided they had no polyuria or ketonuria. The results were striking in that, of patients with a diabetes duration over 15 years, only 9% of the multiple-injection group had nephropathy, compared with 61% of the free-diet group. Nearly a quarter in the strict-control group had had more than 20 attacks of hypoglycaemic coma, compared with only 5% in the free-diet group. None of the eight patients who had been in coma more than 20 times had proteinuria after 25 years and four had normal fundi. Lawrence, like Johnsson, concluded that frequent hypos, a surrogate marker of attempts to keep the blood sugar normal, were generally associated with fewer complications. He added that:

> From my experience the occurrence of 20 comas is carrying hypoglycaemias unnecessarily far.

He also thought that other factors must be involved in the development of complications, writing that:

> Diabetic control, so far as it is possible, can hardly be the whole answer to visual troubles, as there are exceptions in both directions: some, careless and uncontrolled, retain perfect vision; and one of the best-controlled young diabetics I know – my lab man [HR Millar] – went blind from neovascularisation trouble without renal or

vascular complications and his case is one of the major puzzles and disappointments of the first 40 years of my practice.

By the Second World War, it was fairly certain that young thin patients were insulin-deficient and older fat ones insulin-resistant. This was difficult to prove because of the problems of measuring insulin concentrations. In 1947, Evelyn Anderson (1899–1985) and colleagues at the National Institutes of Health in the United States produced rats that were incredibly sensitive to insulin. They did this by making them diabetic with the beta-cell poison alloxan and then removing the adrenal medulla and pituitary gland. These mutilated animals were so sensitive that 0.0001 units of insulin lowered their blood sugar.[22]

Anderson's work was repeated by Joseph ('Ginger') Bornstein (1918–94), who was born in Warsaw and emigrated to Australia at the age of 9. His research career began in 1947 at the Baker Institute in Melbourne, where, according to his own account, he went to the director Basil Corkill with the suggestion that there were two kinds of diabetes and that he might be able to prove this with an animal sensitized by hormonal ablation. In spite of heavy surgical mortality, he succeeded in producing alloxan-diabetic hypophysectomized adrenalectomized rats that turned out to be sensitive to 1/20,000 of a unit of insulin. He was to have continued his studies with Frank Young in Cambridge, but space was not available and he therefore went to Charles Gray's Department of Chemical Pathology at King's – a lucky break because there he met Lawrence, who provided the clinical material. When he tried to measure insulin in humans, Bornstein found that between 0.5 and 1 mL of plasma was needed; unfortunately, giving this volume intravenously to anaesthetized rats often caused death from cardiac failure.[23] He modified the technique so as to carry it out on a relatively stable baseline blood sugar and then found that as little as 0.05 milliunits of insulin lowered the blood sugar. He pointed out that his technique did not measure insulin as such, but only 'the excess of insulin over its antagonists absorbed in unit time'. This was important, because the finding of no insulin could simply mean that, under the test conditions, it was concealed by an excess of antagonists. With Lawrence, Bornstein used his technique to assay plasma insulin in two polar groups of patients: five with newly diagnosed insulin-dependent diabetes had no detectable insulin, while five overweight newly diagnosed elderly diabetics all had measurable levels.[24]

Bornstein's method was far too time-consuming and difficult for routine clinical use. Luckily, clinicians were not clamouring to measure insulin, and, indeed, diabetes remains virtually the only endocrine deficiency disease in which measurement of the missing hormone is unnecessary for diagnosis and treatment.

The disease lipoatrophic diabetes was named and the classical case reported by Lawrence in 1946.[25] The patient was 26 when she presented to the Skin Department at King's with papular xanthomas. She had had diabetic symptoms for 9 months, but otherwise felt well. She was thin and had gross hyperlipidaemia, with a total fat of 6 volume%, which separated as a thick cream on standing. At first, her diabetes came under good control on insulin, but a year later she came back with hepatosplenomegaly, which Lawrence described as introducing 'a new element of interest'. Lipoatrophy developed gradually, so that, 3 years after diagnosis, she had no subcutaneous fat in the face, neck and shoulder girdles. She became extremely insulin-resistant and at one point was treated with up to 1000 units daily for 10 days without developing hypoglycaemia. Ketosis was always absent. One of the most striking features of her condition was the very high metabolic rate, for which a thyroidectomy was performed 6 years after her first presentation, 'with no clear preconception what would result'. In the event, it had no effect, and putting her on thyroxine simply restored her basal metabolic rate to +100%. A year later, her abdominal distention had increased and two large ovarian cysts were removed. Unfortunately, the wound became infected and she died three weeks later.

On looking back through the literature, Lawrence could only find a few similar cases. In 1928, Ziegler from the Mayo Clinic had reported what seemed to be an identical case. This was a 27-year-old woman with total lipodystrophy, gross hepatosplenomegaly, diabetes and a raised metabolic rate. She had 'large brown itching areas all over the skin' but no xanthomatosis or lipaemia. She had apparently given birth to a living child in 1930 and died in 1936.[26]

Lawrence thought that the clue to the pathogenesis of this curious condition was the lipoatrophy and proposed that:

> No fat could be stored in the usual depots and so it circulated in excess and produced lipaemia. The lipaemia depended directly on the level of blood sugar and disappeared repeatedly when the hyperglycaemia was controlled by enormous doses of insulin.

He went on to suggest that there might be a fat-fixing factor or hormone that she lacked. There are now known to be several different lipodystrophic syndromes with varying aetiologies. The acquired form that Lawrence described is called the Lawrence–Seip syndrome.[27]

Haemochromatosis or bronzed diabetes had been described in the nineteenth century. In 1934, Sheldon reviewed 304 cases from the literature and 7 of his own. He noted the very striking sex incidence and wrote that:[28]

> Typically the patient – almost certainly a middle aged man – will present four features, one or more of which may however be absent. These are an enlargement of the liver, caused by a hypertrophic cirrhosis; a bronze pigmentation of the skin, which usually has in addition a peculiar slaty blue or metallic nuance; a diabetes of severe type; and a form of sexual hypoplasia.

Sheldon could only find five definite instances in the literature in which brothers had been affected, and this prompted Lawrence in 1935 to report the family history of one of his patients.[29] He had obtained much of the information by correspondence, but of nine siblings two brothers had definite haemochromatosis and three others may have done. The striking male preponderance led him to suggest (wrongly) that, 'like haemophilia', it was a sex-linked hereditary disease. The next year, he was invited to write an article for the *Lancet* on the prognosis in haemochromatosis.[30] Before insulin, according to Lawrence's reading of the literature, 50% had died of diabetic coma and Sheldon's book gave the average duration of life after diagnosis as 18½ months. Lawrence described 12 of his own patients, of whom 6 had survived more than five years:

> I see no reason to tell these patients they have a fatal disease and think it best, if necessary, to say that their diabetes is complicated by a large liver. The intelligent ones should never hear the words 'bronzed diabetes' or 'haemochromatosis' when perusal of the older encyclopaedias must be unnecessarily depressing.

In 1940, he published a case report in the *Lancet* of a 73-year-old woman: 'the oldest female case of haemochromatosis so far recorded'.[31] Lawrence's final paper on haemochromatosis was in 1949, when he described two new families, as well as 'the only female case I have seen in comparison to 39 males'.[32] Had a referee been asked to look at the paper, he would have noticed that her age is now given as 66 rather than 73 and her blood sugar as 384 mg/100 ml (21.3 mmol/L), compared with 358 mg/100 mL (19.9 mmol/L) in the 1940 paper. It seems that Lawrence had forgotten his 1940 paper, since it is not referenced.

It has been shown in conflicts as far separated in time as the Siege of Paris in 1870 and the Siege of Sarajevo in 1993 that war, and the resulting famine, is 'good' for those with type 2 diabetes. However, war or societal breakdown poses extreme danger for the type 1 diabetic, who is likely to be deprived of a regular supply of insulin. In 1940, Lawrence wrote a short article in the *BMJ* entitled 'Wartime precautions for diabetics'.[33] He pointed out that for severe diabetics (those on more than 30 units of insulin a day):

> Sugar returns as soon as the insulin action is exhausted, even if no food is eaten; acetone bodies rapidly follow, and coma from ketosis may result within a day or two.

Having pointed out that the country had stockpiled enough insulin for two years, he suggested that people on insulin should have a month's ration in case of local supply difficulties. Because of the ever-present possibility of transport delays, people should take their syringe and insulin with them to work even if they did not normally give an injection during the working day. Carrying something to identify oneself as a diabetic was even more important than in peacetime. If their usual brand of insulin was not available, there would be no problem in switching from, say, Boots to Burroughs Wellcome. If insulin was either not available or in short supply, he advised taking the normal carbohydrate allowance but omitting all fat.

Early in 1941, Lawrence wrote to the *BMJ* about panic buying of insulin.[34] National emergencies like the fall of France or the start of the London Blitz pushed up the demand for insulin by 20–40%, which caused people to panic and put demands on their local chemist, who in turn pressurized the manufacturers. There was a national shortage of glass, and Lawrence pointed out that if people using 20-strength insulin switched to 40 units/cm^3, 20,000 bottles per week would be saved. In fact, he thought this was the ideal time to ditch 20-strength insulin, although to make such a change, 'I suppose the *British Pharmacopoeia* and other necessarily slow moving bodies must be concerned.'

Also in 1941, Lawrence noted that many patients following the line ration scheme for their diet had found great difficulty because of the restriction of protein food, and to some extent fat, in the country and advised that increasing carbohydrate and insulin would help to maintain weight. Another annoyance for diabetics was the disappearance of grapefruit and oranges, which 'rounded off many gastronomic corners by supplying tasty bulk with little carbohydrate':[35]

> *Diabetics on low carbohydrate diets must depend more on native vegetables, and they are reminded that freshly grated cabbage, sprouts, celery, turnips and carrots can make appetizing salads when lettuce and tomatoes are not available.*

Unsurprisingly for someone who had diabetes himself, Lawrence had a keen interest in the restrictions imposed by the disease in society. In 1938, with Kate Madders (1884–1974), he wrote an article in the *BMJ* on the employment of diabetics.[36] This began by suggesting that in the minds of the public all diabetics were invalids and that in England a diabetic:

> *cannot enter any Governmental or similar service, is barred from all types of employment which are pensionable, and is liable to find himself discharged when his private employer knows of his diabetes.*

They surveyed 100 clinic patients (75% men) who had been in a job for an average of 5 years. Nearly three-quarters were under age 40, and five out of six were on insulin. Their jobs included gardening, engineering, carpentry, commercial travelling, shopkeeping, office work and domestic work. After the initial period of stabilization, 77% reported having had no time off because of their illness. Lawrence and Madders concluded:

> *We think, however, the survey shows that most treated diabetics are good employees from the health point of view, and hope that the widespread prejudice against their employment may be removed.*

By 1950, the literature indicated that most people with diabetes who were under reasonable medical care had work records comparable to those of non-diabetics. At a seminar on diabetes in industry in Pittsburgh in 1949, Dr Joseph Beardwood of Pennsylvania suggested that:[37]

> *the careless diabetic is also the careless workman and that the diabetic who cooperates with his program will prove to be a conscientious and dependable member of any organisation.*

Nevertheless, he pointed out that the so-called 'graveyard shift' from 11 pm to 7 am was bound to cause trouble and diabetics should be:

> *restricted from hazardous occupations which require them to manipulate complicated machinery.*

One form of complicated and dangerous machinery was the motor car. The 1930 Road Traffic Act abolished the speed limit and introduced an unsupported declaration of physical fitness as the only requirement for would-be drivers. The 1934 Act introduced the driving test, pedestrian crossings and a 30 mile-an-hour limit in built-up areas. In 1946 in the *Diabetic Journal*, the publication of the Diabetic Association and forerunner of *Balance*, it was said, probably by Lawrence, that:[38]

> *It is most unwise for any diabetic, who knows that he does not always recognise the symptoms of hypoglycaemia, to drive a car at any time.*

In a radio broadcast in England in 1948, the doctor narrator said:[39]

> *One thing that must occur to all of us is should diabetics drive cars? I understand the legal position is that diabetics can hold driving licences and do not have to reveal in applying for them that they are diabetics. This puts a great responsibility on them to see that they are not a danger on the road. A few unstable diabetics who are particularly liable to reactions should not drive at all and it's their doctor's business to tell them so.*

In 1948, at the inception of the National Health Service, the *Diabetic Journal* carried lists of diabetic clinics. There were 22 in London, 3 in Birmingham and 3 in Glasgow. What is striking is that most were only held on one half-day each week. By 1953, there were 32 clinics in London and 109 in the provinces. They held about 200 sessions a week and catered to a diabetic population of 200,000.[40]

In 1951, Lawrence suggested setting up special centres for diabetes in London and the southeast of England.[41] The rationale was that:

> *Most general consultants (and their house physicians!) feel that they are ill equipped to deal with diabetics in general wards or afterwards as outpatients. Diabetics themselves crowd to any centre where their problems can be helped or solved.*

He suggested that:

> *In a small centre with some 300 diabetics, the doctor needs one sister trained in diets and insulin and able to teach, a nurse to help her, and a cooperative house-physician. The same team should see the outpatients at their regular visits, at least three or four times a year ... the prime essential is a continuity of personal supervision for months and years. The patients need this, and it pays economically.*

References

1. Deckert T. *H. C. Hagedorn and Danish Insulin.* Herning, Denmark: Poul Kristensens Forlag, 2000.
2. Lawrence RD, Archer N. Some experiments with protamine insulinate. *Br Med J* 1936; **i**: 747–9.

3. Scott DA, Fisher AM. Studies on insulin with protamine. *J Pharmacol Exp Ther* 1936; **58**: 78–92

4. Lawrence RD. Zinc-protamine-insulin in diabetes: treatment by one daily injection. *Br Med J* 1939; **i**: 1077–80.

5. Wilder RM. Recollections and reflections on education, diabetes, other metabolic diseases, and nutrition in the Mayo clinic and associated hospitals, 1919–1950. *Perspect Biol Med* 1958; **1**: 237–77 (p 266).

6. Fletcher CM. One way of coping with diabetes. *Br Med J* 1980; **i**: 1115–6.

7. Lawrence RD. Treatment of 90 severe diabetics with soluble insulin for 20–40 years: effect of diabetic control on complications. *Br Med J* 1963; **ii**: 1624–5.

8. Lawrence RD. Insulin hypoglycaemia: changes in nervous manifestations. *Lancet* 1941; **ii**: 602.

9. Lawrence RD. Hypoglycaemia in road users. *Lancet* 1952; **ii**: 489.

10. Lawrence, R.D., Meyer, A, Nevin S. The pathological changes in brain in fatal hypoglycaemia. *Quart J Med* 1942; **11**: 181–201.

11. Lawrence RD. Prognosis of diabetes in children. *Lancet* 1934; **i**: 807–8

12. Hirschberg J. Über diabetische Netzhautenzündung. *Dtsch Med Wochnschr* 1890; **16**: 1181–236.

13. Wagener HF, Dry TJS, Wilder RM. Retinitis in diabetes. *N Engl J Med* 1934; **211**: 1131–7.

14. Rabinowitch IM. Prevention of premature arteriosclerosis in diabetes mellitus. *Can Med Assoc J* 1944; **51**: 300–6.

15. Lawrence RD. Refraction changes in diabetes. *Br Med J* 1932; **ii**: 1034.

16. Lawrence RD, Levy AH. Vascularisation of iris and cornea in diabetes. *Br J Ophthalmol* 1936; **20**: 198–201

17. Diabetes and the eye. *Br J Ophthalmol* 1943; **27**: 509–13.

18. Lawrence RD. Acute retinopathy without hyperpiesis in diabetic pregnancy. *Br J Ophthalmol* 1948; **32**: 461–5.

19. Lawrence RD. Insulin therapy: successes and problems. *Lancet* 1949; **ii**: 401–5 [The Banting Memorial Lecture of the British Diabetic Association].

20. Lawrence RD. Treatment of 90 severe diabetics with soluble insulin for 20–40 years: effect of diabetic control on complications. *Br Med J* 1963; **ii**: 1624–5.

21. Johnsson S. Retinopathy and nephropathy in diabetes mellitus: comparison of the effects of two forms of treatment. *Diabetes* 1960; **9**: 1–8.

22. Anderson E, Lindner E, Sutton V. A sensitive method for the assay of insulin in the blood. *Am J Physiol* 1947; **149**: 350.

23. Bornstein J. The insulin content of blood plasma. *Diabetes* 1953; **2**: 23–5.

24. Bornstein J, Lawrence RD. Two types of diabetes, with and without available plasma insulin. *Br Med J* 1951; **i**: 732.

25. Lawrence RD. Lipodystrophy and hepatomegaly with diabetes, lipaemia and other metabolic disturbances. *Lancet* 1946; **i**: 724–31, 773–5.

26. Ziegler LH. Lipodystrophies: report of 7 cases. *Brain* 1928; **51**: 147.

27. Martin Seip (1921–2001) was a Norwegian paediatrician who in 1959 described generalised lipodystrophy (without diabetes) in three siblings.

28. Sheldon JH. Haemochromatosis. *Lancet* 1934; **ii**: 1032–6 [The Bradshaw Lecture]. Also: Sheldon JH. *Haemochromatosis*. Oxford: Oxford University Press, 1935.

29. Lawrence RD. Haemochromatosis and heredity. *Lancet* 1935; **ii**: 1055–6.

30. Lawrence RD. The prognosis of haemochromatosis. *Lancet* 1936; **ii**: 1171–2.

31. Lawrence RD. Bronzed diabetes in a woman. *Lancet* 1940; **ii**: 489.

32. Lawrence RD. Haemochromatosis in three families and in a woman. *Lancet* 1949; **i**: 736.

33. Lawrence RD. Wartime precautions for diabetics. *Br Med J* 1940; **2**: 316–17.

34. Lawrence RD. Insulin supplies and wartime economy in prescribing. *Br Med J* 1941; **i**: 251.
35. Lawrence RD. War difficulties in diabetic diets. The line ration scheme. *Br Med J* 1941; **ii**: 118–9.
36. Lawrence RD, Madders K. The employment of diabetics. *Br Med J* 1938; **ii**: 1076–7.
37. Murray AV. Social and economic implications of diabetes. *Ind Med Surg* 1950; **19**: 263–70.
38. Anon. *Diabet J* 1946; **5**: 15.
39. Diabetics at work or on holiday. Reprinted in *Diabet J* 1948; December: 301.
40. Walker JB. Field work of a diabetic clinic. *Lancet* 1953; **ii**: 445–7.
41. Lawrence RD. Regional centres for the treatment of diabetes. *Lancet* 1951; **i**: 1318–19.

CHAPTER 8

Speaking Out: Lawrence and the Diabetic Association*

The Diabetic Association was formed on Lawrence's initiative in 1933 and in doing so he left a lasting legacy. In 1954, it was renamed the British Diabetic Association and then, in 2001, Diabetes UK. The Association aimed to promote and represent the interests of people with diabetes by forging a link between health professionals, patients and carers in an organization that could create pressure for change. In many ways, it extended into the political sphere what Lawrence had learnt from clinical practice – that the management of diabetes was best achieved through a *partnership* between the patient and health professionals.

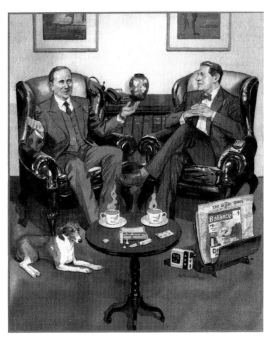

From the 75th Anniversary edition of Diabetes UK. *An imaginary picture of RD Lawrence and HG Wells in conversation as they conceive their 'Association for rich and poor.' The picture shows them surrounded by objects that would come into being over the next 75 years as a result, directly and indirectly, of their vision and endeavours. These include: an insulin kit, non-insulin tablets and some* Diabetes UK *cups, all on the table; a blood glucose meter on the floor; an insulin pump on the arm of Lawrence's chair; insulin pens in both men's breast pockets; a Diabetes UK Careline phone on the bookcase, with the headpiece hooked over Wells' chair; 'Silent Assassin' and 'Measure Up' campaign posters on the wall behind; and, of course, Balance in the newspaper rack, with that all-important edition of* The Times *nestling behind. For good measure, Wells' famous 2/6d (which had been his contribution to the fund for enlarging the diabetic out-patients department at KCH) sits on the table, while, in an even greater flight of fancy, Banting and Best's dog Marjorie, who played such an important role in the development of insulin, listens in quiet approval. (Brian Burns).*

* Much of this chapter has drawn extensively on the published and unpublished work of the BDA's first Secretary General, J. G. L. (Jim) Jackson (1922–2003).

By the early 1930s, the clinic at King's College Hospital was becoming overcrowded and Lawrence asked for further resources. Impressed by the growing fame of the clinic, the hospital authorities agreed to improve outpatient facilities and were sympathetic to a new inpatient ward provided that £800 could be raised through voluntary contributions.

Lawrence wrote to his wealthy patients to raise funds, and, in response, H. G. Wells agreed to a meeting at his home to work out a plan. No doubt at the suggestion of Lawrence, Wells wrote a letter to *The Times* to raise money for improved services at King's. This was a newspaper widely read by the better-off and would give publicity not only to the needs of people with diabetes but also to the services at King's.

In the letter, published on 19 April 1933, Wells addressed readers with diabetes and had no compunction in publicizing his own medical condition. Both he and Lawrence believed that people with diabetes belonged to a special 'cult' and should 'speak out' about their condition, at a time when the diagnosis was feared. By speaking out, both men believed they could encourage others that a normal life was possible and so reduce the stigma attached to the disease. Under the heading 'The select company of diabetics', Wells described the cramped conditions at King's and the sum needed to improve the service. He wrote:[1]

It would be a becoming thing for the elect class of grateful diabetics to whom I appeal to tax themselves for the benefit of our cult. If 40 of us would put up £20 each the thing would be done.

He expressed surprise that there was not already an association:

to watch over and extend this most benign branch of medical science to which we owe our lives.

The £800 was raised within weeks, which encouraged Lawrence and his supporters to take the further step of setting up a Diabetic Association. In November 1933, another meeting was held at Wells's home. The group of 12 included several London-based medical colleagues and the Sister-in-Charge at King's, Miss Wheeler. They agreed to set up an association to support diabetics, with two committees: one to organize the association and another to plan publication of a quarterly journal. Lawrence also agreed to approach medical colleagues to become foundation members: each would contribute £5 to cover the setting-up costs (£265 in today's prices).

In January 1934, at a further meeting, Wells agreed to write a second letter to *The Times*. It was published on 15 February 1934 and in it Wells appealed to his 'fellow diabetics' to support an association, stressing the shared identity among people with diabetes.[2] In the letter, Wells spelt out the philosophy of the association, based on a community of interest. This, he suggested, reflected 'a psychological truth' – the existence of 'latent solidarity of people subject to a distinctive disorder'. He was aware, as was Lawrence, that long-term illness affects how people see themselves and are seen.[3] By speaking out, Wells normalized diabetes, which he described as 'a relatively simple disease to manage'. He argued that, given the new treatments and 'with will power and intelligence, it is ... within the power of the sufferer to keep well'. Both Lawrence and Wells believed that there was something character-forming in the struggle to overcome a potentially stigmatizing condition.

Wells appealed to both altruism and self-interest. He suggested that those who were better off should contribute to a cause that would help 'their poorer fellow sufferers'. People with diabetes had special needs. Children with the disease had to be taught to self-medicate and balance their diet. Poorer people needed financial support and older people might require special accommodation and support. Wells also underlined collectivist values and the advantages of self-help in a community of the like-minded. This would allow 'an exchange of opinions and experiences and in the collective examination of new foods, remedies and treatments' that would be of mutual benefit to all diabetics. He announced that the Association would publish a journal containing scientific articles on new research findings and abstracts of books and articles on diabetes. It would provide a forum for debate and contain a section for readers' letters where problems could be raised and ideas exchanged. A shorter version of the letter was sent to national newspapers with a mass readership to publicize the Association and hopefully to recruit members from a wide cross-section of the public.

In March 1934, at a meeting to elect officials and agree a constitution, it was announced that £240 had been raised from the public appeal.[4] At this meeting of 32 supporters, Wells was elected President and some of the 'great and the good' voted in as Honorary Vice-Presidents. They included Banting and Best, Lord Horder (1871–1955), Lord Dawson of Penn (1865–1945) and Sir Humphrey Rolleston (1862–1944), the last three all former Presidents of the Royal College of Physicians. Lord Dawson was also the personal physician of King Edward VII. Their position was symbolic and intended to add prestige and help with fundraising.

The role of the Executive Committee was to make policy and manage the Association. Although only elected as Chairman officially in 1938, Lawrence, according to Jackson, chaired every meeting from 1934 until his stroke in 1958. The committee included a mix of people from different professions and lay people with experience of living with diabetes as patients or carers. A majority of the Executive Committee were non-medical and included people with useful qualifications in law, finance, accounting and pharmacy. J. P. McNulty (1891–1968), who had diabetes, was an active founder member. He worked in the advertising industry and played a major role in launching and sustaining the Association's journal.[5]

Two other founder members are of particular interest. These were the novelist Hugh, later Sir Hugh, Walpole (1884–1941) and G. D. H. Cole (1889–1959), academic, political theorist and writer of detective fiction, both of whom had diabetes. Cole was an Oxford don and part of the intellectual left. In 1920, he was a supporter of Guild Socialism, a movement that advocated workers' control of industry through trade-related guilds. He believed that[6]

> society is a complex of associations held together by the wills of their members, whose well-being is its purpose ... Society will be in health only if it is in the full

sense democratic and self-governing … This involves an active and not merely a passive citizenship on the part of the members.

The Socialist League, of which Cole was a founder member, was active in the 1930s. It helped to set up local branches, promoted and carried out research, and issued pamphlets, reports and books. It organized conferences, meetings and lectures in schools. It is not known how active Cole was in the Diabetic Association, but his ideas about associative democracy were in accord with those of Lawrence.

The medical members, 12 in all, included diabetes specialists who ran services of a similar kind to Lawrence, such as Otto Leyton (1873–1938) and George Graham (1882–1971). Leyton ran an outpatient service at the London Hospital that was dedicated to treating poorer people from London's East End. Jackson tells us that Leyton treated many patients at his own expense.[7] Graham was a consultant at St Bartholomew's Hospital and had designed the Ladder Diet as a guide for patients. In contrast to the extrovert Lawrence, Otto Leyton was described in his obituary as a reserved and dilettante figure who finished his ward round in half an hour and then 'treated his clerks to an interesting but entirely theoretical discourse', while Graham was a shy, punctilious bachelor about whom an obituarist wrote that he 'might not have been the world's greatest clinician'. In addition, the Executive asked various medical bodies for nominations to a Medical Advisory Committee, the role of which was to advise the Executive on clinical matters and develop policy. It had 40 members, many of whom were clinicians working in London teaching hospitals – a bias that was later to be the cause of resentment.

At the meeting in March 1934, a constitution was drafted by another of Lawrence's patients, the solicitor G. E. Hart. It was to be a non-profit-making organization, with the following stated aims:

- Support mutual aid, promote the study of diabetes, the dissemination of knowledge and the improvement of treatment.
- Safeguard the social and economic interests of diabetics and support international collaboration.
- Develop services such as convalescent homes, educational facilities for children, restaurants and boarding houses
- Develop supplies and equipment.
- Publish a journal.

In 1936, the Diabetic Association was incorporated as a company whose profits were used for the benefit of members. If the association ran into financial problems, the liability of members was limited to 10 shillings. At that time, there was no Charity Commission to regulate voluntary organizations, so the Board of Trade awarded the licence for incorporation – according to Jackson, a time-consuming process. The annual subscription was set at £5 (the annual average income at the time was £192.40[8]).

The membership grew slowly. By the end of 1935, it was 400; by the end of 1936, it was 1676 and by the end of 1938 it was 2130. The Executive found this 'disappointing'.[9] The slow recruitment may have been due to a number of factors that added strength at the time of formation but in the longer run may have inhibited expansion. In the years up to and including the war, the Association was centred on London, as reflected in the membership of its committees. Most of its out-of-London activities were based in the southeast and its members were likely to have been recruited from the better-off.

Nevertheless, from Jackson's history, we know that the needs of poorer people were a major concern to the Executive. Jackson writes that at the time the Association was formed, the outlook for someone with diabetes was bright, but it was clouded by a heavy financial burden.[10] People with diabetes had three main additional expenses:

- The recommended (low-carbohydrate) diet cost more. Cheaper foods such as bread, potatoes and rice were restricted, while foods that could be freely eaten, such as meat, fish, eggs, vegetables and fruit, were beyond the means of many.
- Insulin was also costly: a patient's expenditure could vary from as little as tenpence halfpenny per week to as much as ten shillings and six pence or more, depending on the quality of the insulin and the dose (in 1935, the average income was around £16 per month[11]).
- Syringes and needles could be expensive.

Although the insured could claim insulin on prescription from their panel doctor, some of the more expensive types and better-quality syringes and needles were not always eligible for reimbursement. In the interests of standardizing the benefits paid for by the Approved Societies, the Association approached the National Insurance Authorities to ask them to standardize the type of insulin they would pay for and to include on the list of benefits syringes and test tubes of a better quality. It is not known whether the Association's appeal was successful.

The journal, originally called the *Diabetic Journal* and later *Balance*, was first published in January 1935. The first editor was Hugh Walpole, with Joe McNulty as business manager. It aimed to provide accurate information for lay readers. It described the activities of the committees, publicized fund-raising events and acted as a forum for debate, thus reinforcing a sense of community. Lawrence took a close interest in the *Journal* and, according to Jackson, began jotting down ideas for articles immediately the proposal was agreed. He wanted the *Journal* to provide straightforward practical advice, and, as he excelled in simplifying complex technical information, he wrote much of the copy, although as a matter of policy articles were anonymous. The anonymity may also have related to medical liability. Medical advice could only be couched in general terms, as the exact treatment regime depends on the examination and diagnosis of a particular patient. Moreover, the professional code of ethics prohibited doctors from any form of advertising to attract patients. Writing a popular article might have been construed as touting for patients. Tattersall comments that the *Diabetic Journal* was 'triumphalist'.[12] It tended to focus on people with diabetes continuing to live normal lives and did not discuss the difficulties and complications that could occur. This reflected a choice of style. Lawrence was determined to take a positive approach and encourage others by example.

It was agreed at early meetings that the *Diabetic Journal* should be self-funding through advertising. Initially, the policy of the Editorial Committee was to limit advertisements to medical products such as insulin, syringes and other apparatus. Here the Association was faced with a dilemma. The *Journal* depended on advertising for revenue, but Lawrence wanted to provide accurate information. Diet was a critical element in keeping diabetes under control. Yet information on the precise quantity of carbohydrate, protein and fat contained in food products was often not given on labels or was wrong. By the time the second issue of the *Journal* was published in April 1935, the Executive Committee had developed a policy on advertising food products. Readers were told that the *Journal* would carry advertisements for 'useful and reliable products', but were warned to be cautious. The *Journal* stated:[13]

> *By reliable, we mean products the composition of which is known and published. We warn our readers that these foodstuffs vary greatly in carbohydrate, protein and fat content. The effect on each individual must therefore be considered. Because they are advertised in our pages it does not mean that they can be eaten in unlimited quantities or that they will be suitable for all.*

On a wider front, Lawrence was concerned with advertisements for 'quackery' – remedies he thought were ineffective. Jackson tells us that several products advertised in the national and provincial newspapers were tested by the Association's medical advisory committee and found to be ineffective. Joe McNulty, who had links with the newspaper industry, informed editors of the test results and asked them not to carry advertisements for unproven products.

Through the *Journal*, the Diabetic Association reached a wider audience, and some readers wrote to ask for support to set up local branches. In 1938, as Jackson notes, the Committee discussed the possibility. In 1939, reference was made in the *Journal* to a local volunteer group, but further development was inhibited by the Second World War.[14] A local group was set up in Durham in 1951, and by 1969 there were 76 branches in England.[15] By 2009, there were 400 'local volunteer groups' across the UK, including Northern Ireland.

Over the years, the *Journal* carried articles on research findings, the price of insulin, the availability of services and accounts of discrimination against people with diabetes. When war threatened, there were articles on the implications of rationing and warnings of possible shortages of equipment. It was also a vehicle for publicizing the activities of the Association and providing some form of accountability to members. Announcements were made about the Annual General Meeting; copies of the minutes and the names of the committee members and officers were given. Fund-raising appeals were made, and announcements of new developments at home and abroad were described. Personal stories of people and their experience of living with diabetes, as well as readers' letters, were published to spread information and knowledge and to encourage informal networking. Special clinics and items on government publications and benefits under the national insurance system were also provided. Some issues carried lists of spa hotels in the

UK that provided suitable food for diabetics. Food tables, diet sheets and recipes were regular features.

In the 1930s, another of Lawrence's major concerns was providing evidence to combat prejudice and discrimination against people with diabetes. While health professionals knew that, with insulin, diabetics could live a normal life, this view was not shared by employers and the general public. Regulations in government departments and public companies were discriminatory in terms of both employment and pensions. Tattersall writes that before the Second World War, many employers would not knowingly have taken on someone with diabetes.[16] People on insulin were regarded as a liability, since there was a perception that they might go into a hypoglycaemic coma at any time. Indeed, Lawrence found that some of his patients had lost their job when they were diagnosed as diabetic. Their fear of discrimination encouraged them to hide their disease and inhibited them from asking for time off to attend clinics. To avoid this, Lawrence arranged an evening clinic at King's. In 1938, in an article coauthored with Kate Madders and published in the *BMJ*, he pointed out that diabetics were treated as 'invalids' irrespective of their ability to function normally with treatment.[17] Lawrence and Madders gave the results of a small survey of 100 employed diabetics showing that over three-quarters lost no time due to diabetes after they had been stabilized. Limitations of the survey were acknowledged, but Lawrence argued that the findings showed that an employer's decision not to employ someone who had diabetes was based on prejudice not evidence.

The article pointed out a number of discriminatory practices from an earlier era. A patient with diabetes could not enter a public service that was pensionable. Presumably, this was due to assumptions about morbidity and early mortality. Young male diabetics of working age could also find that they were refused cover by one of the Approved Societies that operated under the National Health insurance scheme. The health insurance that was available through the Post Office scheme provided limited benefits. Whether an article in the *BMJ* could lead to a change in the rules was another matter. One member of the Executive Committee, Joe McNulty, had tried to modify the attitudes of life insurance companies towards providing insurance for someone with diabetes. Most refused any form of insurance cover, while others would only do so at considerably enhanced premiums.

In the 1930s, according to Jackson, motor insurance was unobtainable. However, after the War, it was reported in the *Diabetic Journal* that people with diabetes could obtain driving licences, but the onus was on them to drive sensibly and ensure that their condition was stable. In 1952, Lawrence wrote to the *BMJ* about the risk of drivers having an accident due to a hypoglycaemic attack.[18] This he said, might occur if a person failed to eat the necessary amount of carbohydrate at the usual times, if they took unusually strenuous exercise prior to driving or if they had to change a wheel and then drive. He advised that a way of avoiding an attack was to take extra carbohydrate both before and after any unusually strenuous exercise. A practical solution was to carry a supply of biscuits or sugar lumps for an emergency.

On occasions, the Association acted as a lobbyist for individual children. For example, one mother wrote to the Association in January 1936 to say that her daughter had won a scholarship for secondary education but was unable to take this up because the London County Council (LCC) refused funding on the grounds of a lack of facilities for diabetics. Following informal communications between the Association and the LCC, the decision was reversed. Communication with parents could also identify more general problems that derived from the pre-insulin era. For example, the Association was made aware that many public (fee-paying) schools would not accept children with diabetes. They took action by writing to 45 public or preparatory schools asking for their policy and found that, of these, only two girls' and two boys' schools would accept children with the disease. The Medical Advisory Committee agreed guidelines outlining how children with diabetes could be supported in managing their condition. It is not known whether this led to a modification of the rules.

Given the lack of a comprehensive health service, the services developed by the Diabetic Association raised resources for people with the condition in ways that were innovative and acted as a model for service development in Britain and overseas. In the years before the Second World War, services for children and young people were a priority. The problems facing children with diabetes and their parents were formidable. Insulin prolonged life, but meant a strict regime of diet, injections and urine testing. The LCC was one of the few bodies that had a facility for older children to go for education and treatment. Lawrence had a personal commitment to what he called 'these special children' and he used his networks and political skills to champion their cause.

In 1935, the Association launched an appeal to provide holiday camps. This had been suggested by a member as a good way of allowing children to enjoy being with a community of other diabetics with expert supervision and also of providing respite for parents. Several such camps had been set up in the United States between 1925 and 1932. The Association wanted to buy a permanent site, but this idea was later abandoned. However, two interim camps were held in a private school in Camberley. In the summer of 1936, 20 girls went for two weeks, followed by a camp for 18 boys. Funding was raised through an appeal, and donations were made by the manufacturers of diabetic foods. The camp site was near Windsor Castle and Jackson comments that, for the first camp, 'King George V graciously sent some venison and grouse'.[19] Each camp had a staff of six medical students and adult volunteers. Parents were asked to make a contribution, but children were not refused if their parents could not pay. It is not known how children were selected. The success of this camp led to a subsequent appeal for funds, and further camps were held in 1937. For these, more effort was made to support children who could not afford to provide a holiday themselves.

The need for convalescent homes where people with diabetes could recover from a major illness or operation was another priority. At the time, a few homes were available and some Approved Societies agreed to cover the costs. Unfortunately, these homes rarely had the trained staff or facilities to provide a diabetic diet. The Association approached several London hospitals with a proposal to establish a single centre with a guarantee of a sufficient flow of patients to make the proposition economic. Following negotiations, St Mary's Convalescent Home at Birchington-on-Sea in Kent agreed to accept five women and expand their facilities on the guarantee of 20 patients per year. A nurse trained at the diabetic departments of three London hospitals taught patients how to give injections and control their diet. By 1935, all the beds were fully occupied. A proposal to set up a similar arrangement for men foundered through a lack of support from public authorities and a poor response to a fund-raising appeal. In 1939, with the approach of war, the project was abandoned.

At this time, the special needs of children with diabetes became a priority, and further long-term projects were abandoned. Lawrence was active on a number of fronts. As plans for the evacuation of children were being developed in 1939, the networks of the Association were used to draw up a list of children in London whose parents had agreed to them being evacuated. Hospital departments were asked to send in names and addresses. In the event, only a small number of parents came forward. In 1940, Lawrence also wrote a letter to Charles Best floating the possibility of evacuating children to Canada. He argued that there was a very strong case for getting these 'special children to safe and sheltered conditions'. When Best wired his opposition to the scheme, primarily on financial grounds, the idea was dropped. In 1944–45, with the ferocious bombardment of London by V1 flying bombs and V2 missiles, Lawrence again raised the question of evacuation. At the suggestion of Dr William Allen Daley (1887–1969), then Chief Medical Officer of Health for the LCC, he contacted officials at the BBC and the Ministry of Health to ask for help in providing accommodation for children and elderly and infirm diabetics who had been bombed out of their homes. The BBC agreed, and, in the broadcast, Lawrence appealed to 'the more fortunate diabetics in safe areas' and sent telegrams to many of his patients:

WILL YOU ACCOMMODATE AND LOOK AFTER DIABETIC CHILD EITHER ALONE OR WITH MOTHER, OR ADULT DIABETIC. PLEASE SPECIFY PREFERENCE IN ANSWER.

Following the broadcast, the Diabetic Association acted as the co-coordinating centre for offers and applications. Unfortunately, many replies were negative. By this time, some Britons, including those who lived on a grand scale, were weary of the War. One respondent replied by telegram:

EXCEEDINGLY SORRY EVERY CORNER FILLED IN HOUSE AND ON PROPERTY [with] BOMBED OUT PEOPLE. WILL TRY TO FIND SOMEBODY WHO COULD TAKE THEM. WE HAVE PRINCESS HELENA VICTORIA AND PRINCESS MARIE LOUISE AND STAFF, THREE AMERICAN OFFICERS AND WIFE, THREE FAMILIES WITH 6 CHILDREN. DINING ROOM USED FOR FOUR FEMALE CLERKS FROM WAR OFFICE AS THEY ARE NERVE WRECKED AND COME WHEN THEY CHOOSE. WE HAVE ONLY TWO SERVANTS AND HALL PORTER AND WIFE. I AM MY OWN COOK NOW. WOULD DO ANYTHING TO HELP BUT IT IS OUT OF THE QUESTION. WILL TELEPHONE IF I CAN FIND ANYBODY TO TAKE CHILD.

From early in the War, Lawrence also tried to establish residential units in the London area for children with unstable diabetes. In early 1939, he used his social and medical contacts to enquire about suitable accommodation. The Home Office was cooperative and the Medical Officer at the LCC agreed to help set up a dedicated unit in the Hutton Residential School, near Brentford in Essex, already funded by the local authority. This had accommodation for up to 700 pupils. The aim would be to stabilize the children's diabetes: they would be taught to test their urine, keep to a proper diet and inject their insulin. Lawrence helped recruit a medical officer and in August 1939 the unit was ready. Transport was organized by the Diabetic Association to take the children, and 66 boys and girls were collected from their homes in coaches driven by volunteer drivers. Each child carried a gas mask, a change of clothes, a diet sheet and a syringe. The unit continued to operate throughout the war.[20]

The Hutton unit soon came under pressure to accept children from outside the London metropolitan area. Indeed, there was demand from across the country. Lawrence was aware of this from correspondence to the Association. He noted that

> *from all over the country, from Devon to Lancashire and Durham, the Diabetic Association receives enquiries, mostly from hospital almoners, for somewhere to send children whose diabetes is poorly controlled. There seems to be nowhere.*

He therefore drafted a letter to physicians in cities such as Liverpool and Manchester; under the heading 'Educational Hostels for Difficult Diabetic Children'. He wrote:

> *No doubt you know the problem raised by the difficult and unstable diabetic child. Many of these, either through the severity and instability of their disease, or more often through poor home conditions and lack of supervision, lead a precarious physical existence out and into hospitals for months and their education is often entirely neglected … I have approached the Board of Education. They are most sympathetic to the problem and its solution and have suggested the writing of this letter.*

Aware of practical considerations, he suggested that:

> *the problem is best tackled initially by the physicians of the hospital in charge of such children, and next by their co-ordinated approach to the Medical Officers of the Counties concerned. One difficulty is that there will not be many children in any one hospital area, and co-operation over a wide area will be necessary. We thought a start might be made in such a very populous area as South Lancs., Liverpool, Manchester, etc. Hence this letter to you and a few others, who, we hope, might be interested to help. If not, perhaps you would kindly suggest another name.*

He pointed out that the requirements were not elaborate or expensive. The hostel should be for children of both sexes and of all ages, but mostly from 8 to 14, and the staff should include a matron and a staff nurse trained in diabetic management, with supervision from a physician with access to hospital facilities. Aware of the emotional needs of young children, he commented that the matron should have a 'suitable temperament (motherly!)'.

The letter was sent to 13 physicians, including Professor Norman B. Capon (1892–1975), Professor of Child Health at the University of Liverpool. The two discovered that they had trained together and Lawrence had a willing supporter. Capon agreed to co-coordinate the project in the North of England but, despite his efforts, no units were set up at this time. However, by the end of War, the success of the Hutton unit had become well known both in Britain and abroad. The 1944 Education Act, known as the Butler Act after the then Minister for Education, promised to provide access to a national system of education funded by the state for all children up to age 15 according to age, aptitude and ability. This included provision for children with special needs, and the Hutton unit provided a model for short-term residential care for children with diabetes and was supported by the education authorities. In 1948, the Medical Officer for the Ministry of Education wrote:[21]

Anyone having doubts about the value of a hostel for a minority of diabetic children should visit Hutton. There the boys and girls are taught the diabetic way of life; they test their own urine and, under supervision, inject their own insulin … they lead as free and as normal a life as any child in a public boarding school … they grow into self reliant men and women, fully capable of leading happy and useful lives. Unfortunately, some parents are so foolish that they prematurely withdraw their children from the hostel. The deaths of five children who had been removed from Hutton against advice have been reported.

To meet its obligations under the Act, the Ministry of Education carried out a survey to assess need. This found that there were approximately 1200 diabetic children of school age, of whom up to 150 might benefit from residential hostel accommodation. The Ministry then asked the Diabetic Association to approach organizations in the voluntary sector to provide facilities. Dr Whittaker from Hutton and Miss Holland Rogers approached the Church of England Children's Society, which opened a hostel for 30 diabetic children in Deal in 1949, followed by three others. The National Children's Home agreed to open a further two.

The post-war period in Britain was one of major political and social change. In 1945, the Labour Party's electoral victory brought a government determined to secure protection from poverty and provide access to health, housing and education for the population. Hospitals had already been nationalized as part of the war effort and the National Health Service Act came into force in 1948 and promised access to healthcare free at the point of service. The Bill was fiercely opposed by some doctors and the British Medical Association, but Lawrence was in favour. His main concern was to improve services for patients, and central control was likely to stabilize funding. He had a network of contacts and devoted much of his time to supporting the Diabetic Association and its members. For people with diabetes, the NHS Act brought in a system of registration with a general practitioner and a gateway to hospital services. There was little change initially, but by the 1960s plans were in place to ensure a more equal distribution of services across the country.[22]

The post-war period provided the opportunity for new initiatives by the Association, particularly as its income had begun to increase with the setting up of new branches across the country. In the 1950s, there was a greater focus on research, and plans to provide a dedicated unit for older people were resurrected.

Before the Second World War, the Diabetic Association had awarded grants to clinical researchers who had been recommended by the Medical Advisory Committee, but these were small and for short-term projects. In 1947, at Lawrence's suggestion, the Association agreed to fund an annual lecture in memory of Frederick Banting, who had been killed in an air crash in 1941. The first lecture, entitled 'Recent Canadian Research on Insulin' was given at King's by Charles Best. This was a stand-alone event but the Banting Memorial Lecture later became the highlight of a two-day meeting where diabetes specialists could discuss new developments with financial and administrative support from the Association – a *quid pro quo* was that those attending should join the Association.

In the same year, a substantial sum was donated to the Association by the father of one of Lawrence's patients, to be used to promote research. This increased the number of applications. A subcommittee was formed to allocate grants, but when most were awarded to people working in London teaching hospitals and known to committee members, as the then Secretary General, Jackson, remarked, 'the flames of anatagonism' were kindled.[23] He suggests that Lawrence's dominance of the Association, his high profile with the public following the BBC broadcasts, his extensive social and political networks, his flamboyance, and his occasional high-handedness were resented and undercurrents of discontent surfaced at the annual meetings. In response, changes were discussed and in 1958 agreement was reached to form a separate Medical and Scientific Section of what was by then the British Diabetic Association. The management body of the section was elected to be representative of the range of interests within the specialty, both academic and geographic.

After the war, the Association decided to revive their project for a residential unit for older people. By 1945, there were sufficient funds to buy a property, and this project dominated the work of the Association over the next decade. In 1950, Eastcott, in Kingston-on-the-Hill in Surrey, was acquired and opened in 1953. It was renamed Frederick Banting House and, by the end of 1953, 28 residents had been accepted. By 1959, there were 35. Jackson comments that the Association launched the project as 'enthusiastic amateurs'.[24] The costs of renovation spiralled and additional funds had to be raised. The decision to take a mix of older residents, some of whom were infirm, as well as younger people with chronic diabetes, meant providing facilities for both. When the home was ready, recruiting staff proved difficult, and remained so as staff turnover was high and new recruits needed special training. Managing the accounts was also time-consuming. The financial circumstances of each resident differed: some paid directly for their care or were covered by private insurance. Others were referred by public agencies, but under different funding schemes. Inevitably, some residents found they could not keep up the payments.

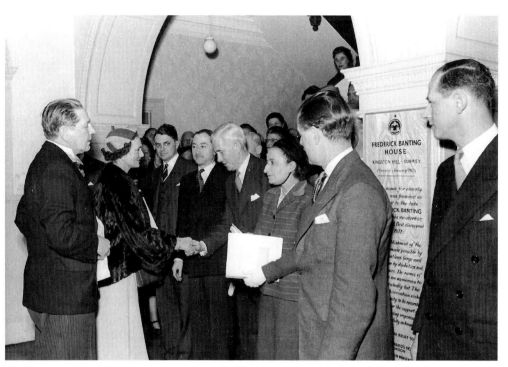

The Opening of Frederick Banting House in 1954. Wilfred Oakley is being presented to HRH the Duchess of Gloucester, Lilian Pearce is holding the papers, and Lawrence is standing behind the Duchess.

The management of Frederick Banting House came to dominate Jackson's life. He coordinated maintenance, oversaw the running of the home and was ultimately responsible for managing the staff and the patients. He made an increasing number of weekly visits over the next years, and eventually took a flat on the premises. He gives a clue to some of the difficulties and says, with a note of irritation:[25]

Whilst the majority of residents accepted the routine of the Home and appeared content, there were others who proved intransigent and argumentative: and additionally failed to follow acceptable hygienic standards. Initially, several complained about poor and insufficient food, but in part this was due to the fact that they had never followed any dietetic instructions in the care of their condition at home.

Despite the difficulties, Frederick Banting House attracted national and international attention, and the model was copied at home and abroad. The Association's Cheshire (Wirral) Branch proposed a second home, and, in 1956, Charles Best House opened with accommodation for 26 residents. However, by 1969, both homes had closed. By this time, health and welfare services were being developed within a planned framework; local authorities were providing more small-scale residential accommodation and had more experience of managing homes in a humane way. Nevertheless, this sector remains a 'Cinderella service' to this day.

In summary, the Diabetic Association, can be seen as a major achievement by Lawrence – a project in which he was closely and enthusiastically involved from the beginning. His passion is evident in an early article for the *Diabetic Journal*, 'The start of it all' giving his account of how the Diabetic Association was founded. He wrote:[26]

> *The Association is a healthy baby and is crying out for food, a wide membership and generous financial support. We don't suppose that one in 50 diabetics in the country have yet heard of its birth. You the readers must broadcast its lusty voice and help it to grow into a useful adult – members and money wanted.*

Lawrence's hopes for the Association were achieved – perhaps even beyond his expectations. Persuading others to support his cause suited his temperament. His desire to help fellow diabetics grew from his own experience, and his ebullience and networking skills were suited to being 'a social entrepreneur' on behalf of people with diabetes. Whittington, a colleague at King's, said of Lawrence:[27]

> *He was a great man because he had one great idea in his mind. Everything is possible for the diabetics. He battled for them, he fought for them and I think that's probably what the patients felt.*

The efforts of the Association to support children were, and still are (for example, summer camps), particularly successful. Residential homes, such as Palingswick House, rescued many a child with unstable diabetes and an unstable home life. The convalescent homes were less successful and their capacity was very limited.

Lawrence's style of leadership had its critics. For example, Tattersall refers to Lawrence's 'paternalism' – but, until recently, paternalism was the professional norm. The patients' movement and a change of attitudes within the profession have placed a greater emphasis on partnership within the doctor–patient relationship.[28] This was what Lawrence always wanted – he knew that successful treatment relied on education and self-control and required doctor–patient cooperation.

With the foundation of the Association, he left a lasting legacy: some 75 years later, Diabetes UK continues to work for diabetics and is a testament to his efforts. In 1940, there were 2,500 members, In 1951, there were 16,000, and by 2012, the membership figure was around 140,000 people with diabetes and 6,000 health care professionals. It employs a staff of 300 and Diabetes UK claims to be the largest voluntary organization in the health care sector.[30] On its formation, the Association was an experiment in social intervention. Its form, with the partnership between patients, carers and professionals was later copied by other groups who aimed to support those with a particular illness or condition in the post-war period.[31]

The Association also encouraged the formation of organizations in other countries, although their structure varied. In 1926, an association for people with diabetes had been set up in Portugal and, in 1938, one for people with diabetes was established in France. In 1940, the American Diabetes Association was founded.

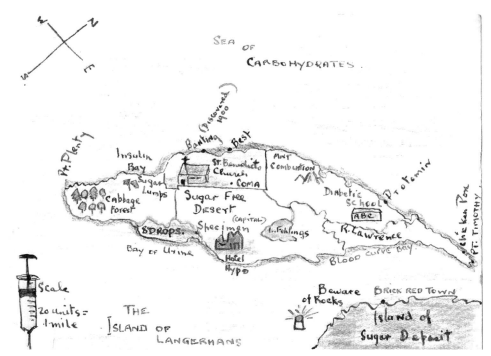

Unpublished post-war sketch for Balance magazine.

In the US the organization was entirely medical, linked somewhat vaguely to 'lay chapters' established in many of the individual States. The Belgian Association, founded in 1942, aimed to protect the interests of Belgian diabetics in wartime. During the 1940s, associations were set up in Sweden, Holland and Australia. The Diabetic Association in Britain was unique in that it brought together patients and clinicians from the outset.

The governing body of the Diabetic Association, in its early stages at least, was what is now termed an insider group.[32] Lawrence chose like-minded people from his various networks to assist in achieving his mission. Many of these owed personal allegiance to him as patients. In the early days, it was driven by his agenda, and the membership was probably biased towards the better-educated. Today, patient and carer groups are expected to be more representative and accountable. However, as his interests widened to the international association, he left the day-to-day management in capable hands.

References

1. Letter and editorial. *The Times*, 19 April 1933.
2. Letter. *The Times*, 15 February 1934.
3. Bury. These ideas were later developed by, for example, Mike Bury in Chronic illness as biographical description. *Sociology of Health and Illness* 1982; **4**: 167–82.

4. Jackson JGL. The History of the British Diabetic Association, Part 1: 1934–38: 7. Unpublished manuscript: (quoting from the minutes of a meeting held on 16 March 1934).
5. Ibid: 5 (quoting from the minutes of a meeting held on 10 January 1934).
6. Cole GDH. *Guild Socialism* (Fabian Tract 192). London: Fabian Society, 1920: Chapter 1.
7. Jackson, Reference 4: 15.
8. This is Money. Historic inflation calculator: how the value of money has changed since 1900. www.thisismoney.co.uk/money/bills/article-1633409/Historic-inflation-calculator-value-money-changed-1900.html.
9. Jackson, Reference 4: 28.
10. Ibid: 1–2.
11. Reference 8 op cit.
12. Tattersall R. *Diabetes: The Biography*. Oxford: Oxford University Press, 2009: 85–6.
13. Jackson, Reference 4: 21 (quoting from *Diabetic J*, April 1935).
14. Diabetes UK. *The First 75 Years Improving Lives*. London: Diabetes UK, 2009: 14.
15. Branches with map. *Diabetic J* 1969; **9**(3): 124.
16. Tattersall, Reference 12: 74–6.
17. Lawrence RD, Madders K. The employment of diabetics. *Br Med J* 1938; **ii**: 1076–7.
18. Lawrence RD. Diabetics and road safety. *Br Med J* 1952; **ii**: 616.
19. Jackson JGL. R. D. Lawrence and the formation of the Diabetic Association. *Diabetic Med* 1996; **13**: 9–22.
20. Ibid: 19.
21. Henderson P. Incidence of diabetes mellitus in children and the need for hostels. *Br Med J* 1949; **i**: 478–9.
22. Webster C. *Health Services Since the War. Volume 1. Problems of Health Care: The National Health Service Before 1957*. London: HMSO, 1988.
23. Jackson JGL. The formation of the Medical and Scientific Section of the British Diabetic Society. *Diabetic Med* 1997; **14**: 886–91.
24. Jackson, Reference 4: 5:34.
25. Ibid: 5:36.
26. Lawrence RDL. Undated handwritten draft for 'The start of it all'.
27. Whittington on his 74 years at King's, in conversation with Dr Peter Watkins and Geoffrey Davies. Unpublished, p15.
28. See, for example, Royal College of Physicians. *Medical Professionalism in a Changing World*. London: Royal College of Physicians, 2005.
29. Tributes to Lawrence. *Balance* (1968) vol.12 No 4: p224–242.
30. *Diabetes UK* (2009) 75 years improving lives. London: BDA.
31. See Baggott R, Allsop J, Jones K. (2005) *Speaking for Patients and Carers: health consumer groups and the policy process*. London; Macmillan.
32. A typology of pressure groups is developed in Whitely PF, Winyard SJ. *Pressure for the Poor*. London: Routledge, 1987. See also Allsop J, Jones K and Baggott R. Health consumer groups: a new social movement? *Soc. of Health and Illness* **26** (6): 737–756.

CHAPTER 9

The 1940s – A Difficult Decade

L awrence was on holiday with his family at 'Saltings' on Hayling Island when on 3 September 1939, the Prime Minister, Neville Chamberlain, told the nation that the country was at war with Germany. Adam vividly remembers sitting round the radio listening to the announcement. Although only six at the time, he froze in the tense atmosphere. The family continued to use the house until 1940, and the boiler room under the stairs was converted into an air raid shelter. Adam remembers seeing air raids on Portsmouth from the roof terrace. Soon after this, the inhabitants were evacuated from Hayling Island. Their furniture was put into storage and the house closed up. The island was used as a decoy to protect Portsea Island. Fires were lit to simulate the bomb damage of Portsmouth and to encourage enemy planes to bomb Hayling, thus protecting the more important military targets in the nearby city.[1]

In common with other families in Britain, their lives over the next six years were subject to many upheavals. 'Saltings' was now out of bounds, their large, comfortable house in Albert Bridge Road was requisitioned, and all their domestic staff left apart from Gwen Amoore, their nanny. In the absence of domestic staff, Anna quickly learned how to master all the household tasks.

The war was a very busy and taxing time for Lawrence and he was placed under considerable strain, being torn in different directions. He needed to continue his clinical work and oversee the safe placement of evacuees with diabetes. He referred to the evacuees not as disabled or handicapped but as 'these special children'. He had worries about the safety of his own family and his frequent separations from them, and needed to offer much support to his patients as they faced difficulties in a London battered by air raids. He continued working at King's College Hospital and in Harley Street, and when his family moved to Wiltshire with Beltane School, he set up a small practice in Bath. Frequently, he drove home in the fog and blackout at the end of a busy day, relying on his one good eye.

He continued to write, and during the war published over 40 articles and letters, including revisions to his books. He served on a wartime Committee for Food Rationing and it was during this time that he met and worked with the government's Chief Nutritionist, Jack, later Sir Jack, Drummond (1891–1952). The two families became friends and Anna was Godmother to the Drummonds' daughter Elizabeth, who was murdered together with her parents in 1952 while on a camping holiday in France.

Charley and Margaret Best in Canada had offered to take Rob and Adam, then aged ten and six, but Lawrence declined the offer in a letter of 20 August 1940, since it was felt that if possible the family unit should be preserved and that Anna and Dan should be included. At this time, Lawrence expected that the boys' school was going to be evacuated to Jamaica, but the plan fell through at the last moment owing to a lack of convoys and the parents' dread of separation.

Although the move to Jamaica did not take place, Beltane School had already established a small country branch on the Shaw Hill Estate in Wiltshire at the time of the Munich crisis in 1938. Two years later, the school at Wimbledon closed, and Anna and the boys moved to a cramped and rather dark house in the small village of Shaw, near Melksham, with Anna's mother, who was by now in her mid 60s. The school took over the large Victorian mansion on the estate. Nearby were the stone-built stables with big loose boxes, stalls, carriage and harness rooms, which enclosed three sides of paved courtyard big enough to hold the entire school. There was a walled vegetable and fruit garden and an old dairy with cowsheds. When the families, including the Lawrences, arrived, they all set to work making a new Beltane. Older pupils worked in their free time with parents and the science teachers to wire and equip the outbuildings with electricity. Others helped teachers dig drainage ditches. Children helped to paint all the outhouses, and they took delight in creating frescos in the dining room. They learnt how to plaster crumbling walls and old corridors and cultivated the vegetable garden to help the school become self-sufficient. The cow stalls were converted to dormitories with bunk beds.

Andrew Tomlinson, the headmaster, was resourceful and innovative when it came to solving problems such as shortage of labour and building materials. He would attend sales everywhere and purchase things to help refurbish and equip the school in its new surroundings. His most successful trip was to Essex, where he recruited five conscientious objectors to work at the school. Later, he bought two railway carriages, which he converted into three double bedrooms. A further purchase was the nose cone of a glider, which was adapted for storage. On one wartime train journey, he met an interesting man and, with no Board of Governors to consult, appointed him as a maths teacher on the spot.

Anna and the three boys were very much a part of the new Beltane. Anna took on a pastoral role and gave valued support to the traumatized refugee children. The boys' classrooms were in the converted stables, with mangers still intact. The jackdaws which had inhabited the deserted stables were quite happy to be adopted as pets by the children when they moved into the converted buildings. Eleven-year-old Rob actively helped in the conversion and decoration programme and Anna taught music and dance. A Hungarian pilot who was stationed at an air force base near Melksham was walking near the school when he heard a pianist practising. He tentatively approached this kindred spirit and, before long, they struck up a partnership and gave many concert performances to the school on Sunday evenings, in which Anna participated. Adam remembers Anna accompanying one particularly brilliant violinist who was a parent at the school, playing Beethoven's Spring Sonata, throughout the slow movement of which his father's eyes streamed with tears.

The Lawrence boys were involved in full-scale productions of Shakespeare plays staged in an outdoor theatre that had been constructed in the school grounds.

There was also a theatre in a converted barn, with a stage, lights, flats, a proscenium arch and raked seating for 100 people. Joan loved immersing herself in drama and she was the driving force behind the plays. Ernst Bulova produced the operas, including *The Marriage of Figaro*, with the school orchestra.

The boys were taken off with their sketchbooks on bike rides to nearby Bradford-on-Avon, and also visited various Wiltshire churches to learn something of architecture. All three boys developed a lifelong interest in church art and architecture, which was first fostered at Beltane.

There was a USAAF unit nearby, and local residents were encouraged to offer hospitality to the servicemen. Anna caused the village net curtains to twitch by inviting a tall, very good-looking black private to the family home. The invitation turned out to be an inspired decision, since he was a jazz pianist from the southern states and with him she learned to play boogie-woogie.

Anna's mother lived with the family at Shaw during the War. She helped with the distribution of orange juice and cod liver oil for the families in the village and took on a welfare role with the land girls who were billeted with local farmers. The boys have very fond memories of their grandmother during the War. Dan recalls how as a small boy she would take him to school each morning and deposit him in the playground – although he always tried to arrive back at the house before his grandmother to avoid being subjected to the Montessori practice of drawing letters in damp sand, since he hated his hands becoming unpleasantly gritty. Gan, as Anna's mother was known, kept the boys motivated throughout this period by giving them small, carefully chosen 'awards' on the completion of domestic tasks. The boys wrote to their father regularly, which must have provided a welcome break for him in the busy working day. Six-year-old Dan gave a concise account of his day and showed how he was honing his entrepreneurial skills by running a small shop, pulling his weight in the wartime household and coming to terms with the repetitious nature of a child's routine:

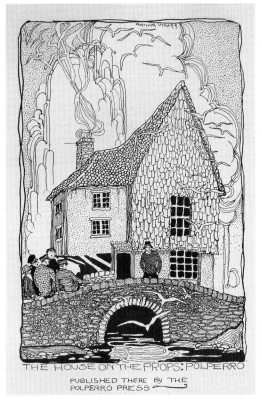

The House on the Props: Polperro

> *I run and slide up to school and I do my lessons and slide back home have my dinner do my reading then I slide back to school more lessons slide home and attend to my shop then have supper then see if any person wants to buy anything then muck around with*

a pack of cards then have my wash and go to bed and then go to sleep after 11 hours of sleep then I get up and have my breakfast and then I feed the hens then I do it all again. Dear Love from Dan

Gwen Amoore, the family nanny, married Anna's brother Tim in 1940 and she lived in the other half of the Lawrence's semidetached house while her new husband served in India. She looked after the boys when Anna went to visit Lawrence in London. Anna took the boys to Cornwall in August 1940 to stay in a rented house at Polperro known as the 'House on the Props'. Despite the idyllic setting for their holiday, she was missing her husband desperately:

Beloved Robin,

Today is Friday and I'm sitting on a marvellous part of the coast – about 2 miles beyond Bedruthen steps – in a place called Porth Mere. It's very wild and solitary and rather beautiful. At this moment the boys are rounding the headland with delighted faces and now they have announced that they saw a seal in the water. We had been told that these creatures are seen round here sometimes. They regard this as the high spot of their trip – earlier in the day we bathed in a marvellous large natural swimming pool in the rocks on an island – where Rob dived in it was probably about 20 feet deep and after half way it gradually sloped upwards into a lovely white sandy bottom with finally a mere paddle out onto dry rocks. So Adam happily practised his breaststrokes and succeeded in making his way backwards too.

You don't say what you think about my going back with you that Monday. I know I would feel it almost unendurable to arrive on Sat eve and only get one clear day with you after all these weeks of separation. What about a flat in the mews and then when the raids begin and Bernal[2] seems to think they will eventually. You could let yourself into the clinic by the side door – but I wonder, would you? Better to go on trying for McCrea's flatlet. Shall I go back to living in London – I think perhaps you need looking after more than the children – Gwen could look after them and live rent free with us.

Dan won't 'need' me very much longer and I could come back for holiday spells. This war may drag on for years (Bernal says) and we'll all be stuck more and more where we are – and I want to be joined to you please. The ties and bands of love, of family of children of home – all very difficult stretched this way and that, but strong and durable, the best quality elastic. Now to sleep after I have looked at some examples of art in the USSR.

Anna and the boys had moved into some converted stables with other Beltane families. The stables were infested with fleas, who lived on the hordes of cats. She finished her letter with a description of how she was waging her own personal war against these fleas:

Rob fondles the cats and never gets a flea on him, but they just come hopping on to me. I can see them doing it. There must be something about me! X Sweetabel ever X

Anna did not move up to London, but continued to live with the children in Shaw for the rest of the War. Her anguish at her continued separation from her husband resurfaced in a note scribbled in pencil on a card from Waterloo Station in April 1944:

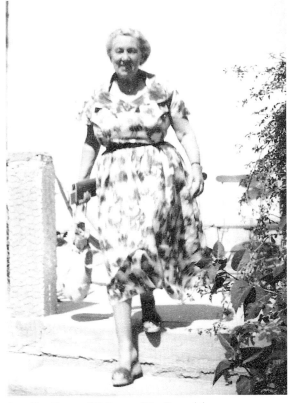

Somehow I didn't like saying goodbye to you at all this morning. You looked so very Bonnie Robinish and smiling – and how much I love you came over me in a wave and it quite engulfed me and for a moment and I wanted to run after you and say, 'don't let's be parted so much.'

She hoped he would have a restful weekend, but she very much wished 'we could all be together'. The letter was signed to her dear one 'my true and only love'.

Joan Tomlinson of Beltane – 'Mrs Tommie'.

In the summer of 1946, Charley Best came over to visit the Lawrences in Wiltshire and wrote to his wife Margaret giving a closely observed description of family life with them:

Robin and I have had several long talks on the problem of diabetes and I have enjoyed it immensely. He makes a better attempt to keep up with experimental work than any other clinician I know. The boys are most interesting – Rob (17) is about Sandy's build and weight. He has matured mentally rather slowly and is still more boyish than Sandy in many ways. He is undecided what to do after he finishes his school. He may be called up for military service for 18 months or two years. If he is not, he will have great difficulty getting the University he chooses. Adam (13) is a very well balanced lad and is going to be a particularly good looking man. He is artistic and tolerates Dannie (10) remarkably well. Dan is at a bad stage. He uses various methods to make his presence known and fully appreciated. If more gentle means fail he takes a kick at Adam. Robin said Dan is going to be a financier and look after us all. Dan, 'I won't be looking after Adam'. Dannie as I wrote before is really a very nice fellow. Anna has been doing all her own work over the holiday but has a cleaning woman who will come almost every week day.

The sister-in-law, the nanny who married Anna's brother lives with her little girl Mary in the other half of this double cottage. She apparently takes responsibility for the Lawrences when Anna goes up to London with Robin. Robin needs care. He had a sharp insulin reaction last evening when the supper was not ready quite as soon as he expected. Anna noticed it before Robin did and it took quite a lot of sugar to restore him to normal.

Lawrence maintained his personal and professional connection with H. G. Wells. In a pre-war letter dated 1 July 1937, Wells, then aged 71, wrote:

My dear Lawrence,
Could you come to lunch with me on Tuesday or Wednesday next and have a professional talk. The situation is this. I think dropping all anodynes and medicaments, bucking myself up with Castor syrup and doing high frequency, has made the arm bearable and usable. But it still aches. The general health is still there. Cumberbatch is going on with the diathermy [heat treatment] but I think that now is the time to take up the general state of the blood, and I feel that you're the keenest and best man for that. Have I any excess of uric acid, sugar – any deficiencies – and if so do we need a new set of rules for diet & drink? Considering the fact that I am a lightweight so to speak, do I take liberties with cocktails, vodka, brandy: have I bad habits? And so forth?
Yours, HG

There are no records describing Lawrence's treatment of Wells, but he kept in close touch, not only as a patient, but also as a friend. In later life, Lawrence recalled visits to Wells, who was nearing the end of his life:

March, 1944. Of course, tired, old, slow and ill physically and equally so in mind. He really cannot think nor express himself the last few weeks: would start a sentence, stop, search for what he began to say, lose it and start again, very disturbed and worried by the state of the world and the disorder in all the ideals he had worked for.

22nd March, 1944. I found him shaving but still with half a beard on him and soap in his ears: every move in the slowest of slow motions but determined to finish everything and remove the last bit of soap from ears with a twisted corner of towel. He had had a bad night: a heavy raid from 1–2 am had awakened him. He had got up and worked and then gone back to an uneasy bed with 'ideas' spinning in his head. 'I am doing quite a lot of work. There are things I must tidy up and leave in order before I pay my account.'
I suggested, as before, that he left London and the bombing to have good nights. 'I can't', he said: 'The Roman Catholics would say I was afraid.'
I watched his reflection sadly in the mirror, a tired, sagging, thinning face. But one bright spot. I heard him muttering 'You doctors, you awful doctors', and then to me, with a little Wellsian chuckle 'You will be just like the Nanny who said "Go and see what little Johnnie (that's me) is doing and tell him not to." '
But when I left it was, as always: 'Bless you, come again soon.'

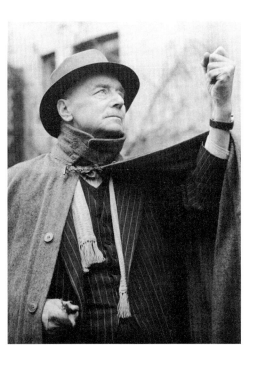

From Lawrence's collection of H. G. Wells memorabilia: 'To Robin Lawrence, to show how we feel about objective professionalism and anti-scientific methods. H. G. Wells'.

Fourteen months later, on 7 May 1945, Lawrence noted:

Short visit to HG about 6.45 pm. My usual four loud taps on his door; a feeble 'come in', and then a stronger 'Hello, Robin'. Found him in his sun parlour with huge panama hat with widely wavy brim, dark glasses and doing, as often, the Times Crossword. *I told him that apparently surrender had come fully and the fighting in Europe was over. There was no response in his tired face or general attitude – perhaps he already knew but had never found him listening to the news. The only remark he produced was that 'now the vested interests will be all over us again'; and 'these must be fought' or some such phrase. A very fixed and very old mind, conditioned by a very feeble and very tired body: but the mind had been similarly fixed (I've always thought) before the bodily vigour so greatly faded.*

His cerebration was dull and I tried the thing that interests me always and him sometimes, of word derivations. 'Wiseacre' was my puzzle and when he suggested, rather feebly, 'wise' with a Latin ending, I thought he might be right. The subject faded (the dictionary proved us both wrong as I found on coming home) and we passed to his bowel problems. I had to search out in his top drawer downstairs his daily diary of such events: times of happenings from 1.00 am etc., and ¼, ½, 1 (full action) or ⅛, merely a fart! Pitiful to me.

10th August 1945. Semi-drowsing in bed. We somehow wandered onto the Atomic Bomb. 'They won't believe it that man can be destroyed and disappear – just can't believe it. I said it would happen, what, some 50 years ago, but it seems impossible to everyone – that man, including themselves, is to disappear.' What did I think? I said that I was perhaps an ostrich with my head in optimistic sand. He said: 'You're not a stoic yet, but something always turns up to make every reasoning man a stoic. Why are you not? What is your optimism?' I said that I wanted widespread better material conditions for the skin and belly which were improving at least here, and besides this, wanted freedom to pursue any whim of mental interest including the arts and beauty. 'You're certainly not a stoic yet', he said. He was less violently in despair than previously about the unreasonableness of man – less violent because so weak.

4th June, 1946. 6.30 pm. Saturday, breathing short and fast before his fire; dying away it was, like him, and though he had moved the guard, I had to pile the wood, as bend and poke he could not. One eye inflamed with conjunctivitis – I gather his anti-itch spirit had dripped in! And so, upright and brave enough, he panted and dozed.

By way of conversation I asked him if he did his Times *Crossword – an inveterate habit. 'No', he said, 'It is too hard work.' 'So you just sit and contemplate', I asked. 'No, I am a complete void, waiting for the end.' No self pity, no emotionalism, a plain statement of realised fact with not enough energy (oxygen) to care. But brave and upright and carrying on what habits he could. And a week ago, he said: 'I wish I could be 20 years younger or else finish soon': this a propos of more he wanted to write about, a world social order he wished to tidy up a bit more.*

After his last visit to Wells, when 'he refused any medical examination as a waste of time, which it certainly was', Lawrence drove back to King's:

with tears in my eyes at having – rightly it turned out – seen the last of dear HGW whom I, like so many others, had come to love as well as admire. My nerves were greatly jangled and I snapped inexcusably at some of the hospital out-patients, and after some nights of insomnia, I even snapped at my dear and sympathetic wife who said 'Robin, you are past the end of your London Doctor tether. Go and catch trout.' So I went to the Hampshire Test, slept on a farm, put myself under the fishing charge of the good water-keeper, Mr. Mott of Longstock, slept from exhaustion and knew I had recovered my balance when on losing the best trout, probably 5 lb., I said 'damn' only once.

Hugh Clegg, then Editor of the *BMJ*, had cause to write to Lawrence later on another matter, but added as a postscript:

I knew your old patient and co-founder of the Diabetic Association – HG Wells – very well indeed. I remember him telling me about his own diabetes and his saying something like this: 'Robin Lawrence is a good scientist as well as a good doctor.'

J. B. Priestley described Wells as 'a man whose word was light in a thousand dark places'. Lawrence's admiration for Wells was expressed in more specific terms when he bought, at the sale of Wells's belongings, a bust of Voltaire (which turned out to be by Houdon), and the *Webster's Dictionary* to which they had so often referred was bequeathed to him.

In the autumn of 1946, Lawrence himself was suddenly taken ill with pneumonia and was admitted to the London Clinic. A nursing sister on duty recalled that he had just given himself some insulin when he vomited and became worried about not being able to retain food: 'Someone managed to find a grapefruit for him (such fruits were difficult to obtain at that time).' This he quickly ate and recovered well. However, his illness was severe and it transpired that he was allergic to the penicillin with which he was being treated. He needed a long convalescence and went with Anna to Portugal for several weeks.

After the War, Lilian Pearce organized the rental of a maisonette for the family on the top floor of a house in Devonshire Place that was a few minutes walk from Lawrence's consulting room in Harley Street. The rooms were small with low ceilings and there was no garden, but it was very conveniently located, with all the facilities of central London on the doorstep and ten minutes' walk from Regents Park. Anna would practise her piano in the early evening so that Lawrence could be undisturbed to read and do his writing in the living room after supper. They kept a splendid radio-gramophone in the room for playing their large collection of records and they would also listen avidly to the cricket commentaries. They lived there for 12 years.

In the late 1940s, Lawrence also bought a half share in Warren Court Farm with his colleague from King's, John (later Sir John) Peel (1905–2006). The farm had fishing rights on the Test and Lawrence particularly enjoyed an annual holiday there in September.

In 1947, Lawrence published a book *Happiness and our Instincts. A Doctor's View of Human Needs*,[3] which was reviewed in the *Eugenics Review* by Carlos Paton Blacker (1895–1975),[4] General Secretary of the Eugenics Society. It may come as a surprise that Lawrence was a member of the Eugenics Society, since the whole concept of eugenics has been discredited by the Nazi programme of enforced sterilization and later extermination of the 'unfit'. The British society was founded in 1907 against a background of concern that the population was degenerating and that the birth rate had fallen among the most desirable members of society. This, it was thought, would put the British Empire at a disadvantage in future wars. During the 1920s and 30s, when the society had between 600 and 700 members, many prominent politicians flirted with eugenics, which Donald Mackenzie argues was the ideology of the professional middle class.[5] The membership was mainly doctors, scientists and writers. Thus, it included presidents of the Royal College of Physicians such as Lord Platt, Russell Brain, Lord Dawson, and Sir Humphrey Rolleston. John Peel was also a member, as were the birth control campaigners Margaret Sanger, Marie Stopes and Margaret Pyke. The leading light of the society was Carlos Paton Blacker. In an article in 1937, he defined the aim of eugenics as being to 'promote the fertility of people with socially valuable inborn qualities and to discourage that of persons with the opposite qualities'.[4] He admitted that it was not easy to define such valuable qualities, but he tried to persuade the government to introduce voluntary sterilization. The utilitarian argument was that if the unfit were sterilized, they would not need to be kept in expensive sex-segregated institutions and would have the opportunity to marry but not reproduce. Blacker was unsuccessful, but it is worth noting that during the 1930s the United States, Sweden, Norway and Finland all introduced compulsory sterilization.

In his review of Lawrence's book, Blacker wrote:

Lawrence, one of the world's leading authorities on diabetes, a valued member of the Society's Consultative Council, and twenty-five years ago my best man, is a humanist. 'I should define happiness,' writes Lawrence in his stimulating little book, 'as a state of satisfaction of our instincts, a full and satisfying response and reaction to instinctive impulses and forces.'

Blacker noted that:

the book is devoted to the argument that there are four such instincts, of which three are 'more strictly individual' than the fourth. The three individual instincts are those concerned with self-preservation, sex and power; the fourth is the herd instinct. The individual attains happiness by the balanced and harmonious satisfaction of these four instincts.

Blacker's review continued:

But these instincts may clash. In particular, the instinct for power presents difficulties: for it 'has been and is the chief cause of human strife and the chief danger to widespread happiness.' (The dictum that 'all power corrupts and absolute power corrupts absolutely' is duly quoted.)

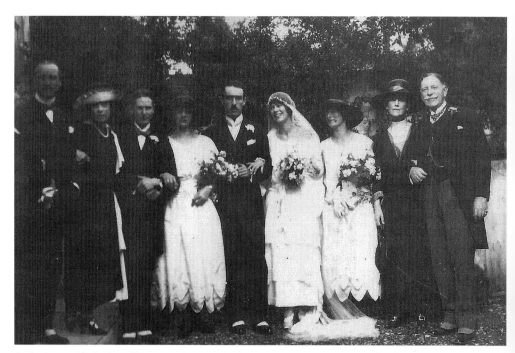

Carlos Paton Blacker's wedding to Helen Maud Pilkington in Florence in 1922. Lawrence is third in from the left.

Hence, wrote Blacker:

> *Dr. Lawrence is confronted with an ethical dilemma. The instinct for power, which leads to strife, must be restrained by the herd instinct which takes account of the needs and claims of others.*
>
> *Various solutions of this dilemma are possible. The obligations which a more pious generation were due to God may today be idolatrously rendered to a corporate state or to a leader. Over more than a sixth of the world's surface (counting the Satellite States), a theocentric system has been, replaced by a tyranocentric. But Dr. Lawrence abhors dictators and his argument leads him (so one may think without the compulsion of dialectical logic) into the safe pastures of liberal democracy. The ethical solution of the dilemma, the necessary, compromise between the power and the herd instincts, are found in the principles of tolerance and liberty. 'The minimum of restraints and laws, written and unwritten, should be imposed, the minimum to safeguard the common rights of others and ourselves. Apart from such restrictions, personal liberty and freedom, permission to differ should be allowed and is necessary for the development of individual happiness.' The rights of children are treated as especially important.*
>
> *Dr. Lawrence's book will therefore be mainly acceptable to rationalists, sceptics and humanists who are also liberals and individualists. Though written in a spirit of humility and without dogmatism, it contains passages about how religious and mystical feelings arise from the natural limitations of the human brain, about the experiences of nuns and about the probable non-existence of free will which may provoke dissent in some readers.*

Blacker ended:

> *At this point my review might fittingly conclude. But there protrudes from my rounded impression of Dr. Lawrence's thesis a sort of jagged interrogation mark which somehow looks, to the eye of the mind, like a baited fish-hook. Dr. Lawrence throws into a chapter on 'existing social structures' an arresting observation which seems to run counter to his general argument. Here it is: 'Judged by the standards of instinctive happiness, the majority of those with power and riches get far less out of life than we might expect … The life, too, of the womenfolk is often empty and unsatisfied, and the idle rich are the unhappiest and most discontented stratum of society I know.' Really? Why? The rich surely have plenty to eat; their sex lives are freer then most; their appetites and material needs are abundantly satisfied; they have the power conferred by wealth; and their herd, social instincts have much latitude.*
>
> *According to this book's formulary one would surely expect that the generous fulfilment of the four primary instincts would lift rich and idle women into a state of enduring happiness amounting to bliss. Yet they constitute the unhappiest and most discontented stratum of society that the author knows. Why? Gem-like, a blue bird seen to flutter momentarily into the outer confines memory.*

Perhaps the problem of happiness is a little more complicated than Dr. Lawrence's simple thought useful analysis suggests.

The Bests were in England in 1949 attending a celebration dinner of the BDA, and Margaret recorded in her diary:

Robin Lawrence spoke on the care of diabetics in England in wartime. Robin looks so young and has so charming a manner. He referred to his own diabetes and the fact that he has taken insulin for 25 years. He said he had no intention of getting any of those awful things – gangrene etc. that the doctors talk about. I think he said that he planned to attend the 50th anniversary (of the BDA). He was very fluent and clever and witty too.

We Saw These Shows...

A CRITICAL REVIEW OF RECENT PROGRAMMES *by Austin Welland*

Televisin weekly [Dec. 10]

Credit for the best performance of the week goes, for once in a way, to a man who does not claim to be an actor. After the opening programme in the " Matters of Life and Death " series had fallen extremely flat, the second demonstrated what really could be done with this subject, thanks largely to the magnetic personality of Doctor R. D. Lawrence, whose patent enthusiasm for his life work was at once communicated to the viewer.

Even if, like myself, you were only casually interested in diabetes, you could not fail to know considerably more about it by the end of the programme. Doctor Lawrence's enthusiasm is so infectious that he should be invited to return to Alexandra Palace and talk about any other subject in which he happens to be interested.

Rare Bird

This programme avoided the mistakes of its predecessor; the laboratory demonstrations were cut down to a bare minimum, and contrived to hold the interest, and the interpolated studio scenes were brief and to the point. Professor Best, one of the discoverers of insulin, also proved an engaging personality, and his short talk was easily understandable to the layman.

Now that the producer and script writer have hit upon the right formula for this type of feature, let us hope they will continue to profit by it. But they will not easily discover another Doctor Lawrence.

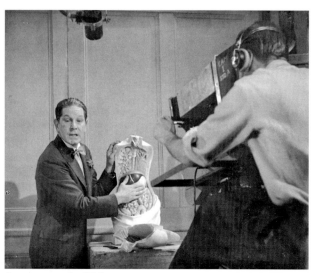

Lawrence on the BBC.

In November 1949, Lawrence featured in a television programme, 'Matters of Life and Death'. It was received with critical acclaim. Lionel Hale in the *Spectator* wrote:

> *It was explained by Dr. R. D. Lawrence, of King's College Hospital, one of those rare people who, by sheer force of personality, come fairly bursting out a television screen into one's drawing room. … in general, it was a triumphant parade of television's potentialities in the documentary field.*

Another review recorded:

> *Now that the producer and script writer have hit upon the right formula for this type of feature, let us hope they will continue to profit by it. But they will not easily discover another Doctor Lawrence.*

These cuttings were kept in Lawrence's scrapbook, and he added, 'Ha Ha!'

References

1. Sharp D, Rendell S. *Connell, Ward & Lucas: Modern Movement Architects in England 1929–1939*. London: Frances Lincoln, 2008.
2. J. D. Bernal (1901–71), referred to by his friends as the Sage of Science, was a friend of the family.
3. Lawrence RD. *Happiness and our Instincts. A Doctor's View of Human Needs*. London: C & J Temple, 1947.
4. Blacker PC. Eugenic problems needing research. *Eugen Rev* 1937; **29**: 181–7.
5. MacKenzie D. Eugenics in Britain. *Soc Stud Sci* 1976; **6**: 499–532.

CHAPTER 10

International Affairs

The greatest thing we have done is to start new movements and get them paid for by other people.

R. D. Lawrence

From 1926 to 1950, an increasing number of national diabetes organizations were founded and many had consulted with the British Diabetic Association and Lawrence for guidance. The increasing impetus towards an international gathering was spearheaded by Professor J. P. Hoet of Belgium (1899–1968), who, like many others, travelled to Toronto to work with Charles Best, and on to Boston to come under the influence of Dr Elliot P. Joslin. In June 1949, 75 patients and doctors from 11 different countries gathered in Brussels for the first international symposium on diabetes, which was unique in that lay diabetic patients were also included – not without some opposition. The lay participants were excluded from the strictly scientific sessions held over two days. But, during the first day, there were talks from lay colleagues on different social aspects of living with diabetes, and ample opportunity for the laymen to exchange ideas and ideals. Lawrence and Hoet were the principle leaders, and Best and Joslin were among the honoured guests. Among the others was M. Maurice Paz, the President of the French Diabetic Association, a redoubtable lawyer and member of the French Socialist Party (and former member of the Communist Party), who vigorously upheld the rights of the lay diabetic to be heard.

Such was the enthusiasm for this new concept of integrated meetings of lay diabetics and their medical advisers that plans were put in hand for a further meeting in the following year, to be held in Amsterdam, organized by Hoet and Dr Fritz Gerritzen, another of those who had been to Toronto. On 23 September 1950, a number of lay and medical delegates met in Amsterdam to put down the foundations of the International Diabetes Federation (IDF). Lawrence was unanimously elected as the first President, a position he held with distinction until 1958. He relished the opportunities for international exchange of ideas that this body provided, but became increasingly disenchanted with the political bias that pervaded its activities. Hoet (Belgium), Paz (France) and Dr Howard F. Root (United States) were elected Vice-Presidents, and Best (Canada) and Joslin (United States) were appointed Honorary Presidents. Gerritzen (Holland), the first Secretary/Treasurer of the Federation, engaged the services of Mr Pieter Duys, a man of great charm and dedication, as Executive Secretary. Plans were made for the First International Congress, to be held in Leiden, Holland, in 1952, at which both medical and lay representatives of national diabetes associations were to be present.

The first IDF Congress, organized by the Dutch Diabetes Association from 7 to 12 July 1952 was almost certainly the first occasion on which doctors interested in a specific disease met with patients afflicted with that disease to formally discuss their mutual problems. It was a considerable success; 241 representatives from 20 different countries attended, most being physicians or scientists, since laymen had great difficulties in raising the necessary funding. Both Honorary Presidents, Charles Best and Elliott Joslin, attended, the former giving one of the plenary addresses. In addition to 47 medical/scientific papers, there was also a medico-social section, in which 16 papers were presented, establishing a precedent that has been followed in all subsequent congresses; a mixture of lay and medical interests. Joslin spent many hours on ancestry tourism, as he was keen to visit the places from which his Puritan forebears had come.

A formal banquet was held on the first night of the congress, but the celebrations on the two following evenings were informal. Best, Lawrence and Professor Lukens sang a few college songs, and Fritz Gerritzen's daughter Viveka played a classical flute sonata, accompanied by Anna Lawrence.

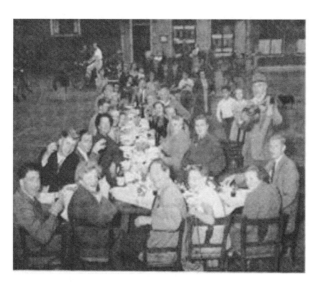

Lawrence taking the chair at a very informal dinner during the first IDF Congress in Leiden, 1952.

Medical students at Leiden assisted with the congress, and Lawrence invited them to a dinner on the last night in a small restaurant, which was quickly filled to overflowing. Margaret Best recorded in her diary that the students carried tables out under the trees in the middle of the square in front of St Peter's Church. Before dinner, Charles Best had taken a ride round the square on the back of a little boy's bicycle. A uniformed policeman joined the gathering, along with the pipe-smoking Chief of Police in a brown suit, who then drank a glass of wine. A photographer came from the local paper, as there had never been a dinner party in the local square before. They moved back into the restaurant for coffee – and more singing.

> *Charley led* Alouette *very capably. Robin sang a Highlands song and we all joined in the chorus by holding our noses in imitation of bagpipe music. We signed our names on the labels of the wine bottles which the students carried away.*

When the Bests left, the students formed an archway, holding up the bottles for them to go under.

Lawrence, and his chief ally Hoet, believed that the ideal diabetes association was one in which doctors and patients worked together for the benefit of the diabetic community, and this was enshrined in the Constitution of the IDF in that the official representation in the General Council was one lay and one medical delegate. But, in fact, few national associations were able to abide by this ruling – partly for economic reasons, but also because not all of them were the hoped-for mixture of doctors and laymen. The American Diabetes Association, for instance, was an entirely medical and scientific organization with no lay affiliation; although they overcame the matter of a lay delegate by appointing their Executive Secretary, J. Richard Connelly, as their non-medical representative.

In January 1953, Lawrence and Anna were busy preparing for a four-month trip to Australia and New Zealand. At one point before the trip, he was anxious that it might not go ahead, as Australian legislation prevented people with diabetes from taking up permanent residence there. A letter from the High Commission of Australia in October 1952 reassured him that the regulation would not apply to him. Lawrence was to be a key speaker at the inaugural meeting of the Victoria Diabetic Association in Melbourne. The couple set sail from Tilbury on 14 January, only to return the same evening as their P&O liner the *Strathmore* broke down an hour after leaving port and had to be towed back to Gravesend for repairs, which took a week. Lawrence probably recovered quickly from the sense of anti-climax and would have appreciated a clear diary to allow him to get ahead with the new book he was writing: *Clinical Medicine: Some Principles of Thinking, Learning and Teaching.*

Once the ship had been repaired, they set sail. The *Strathmore* was used as the India and Australia Mail service and called at Southampton, Gibraltar, Naples, Port Said, the Suez Canal, Aden, Bombay, Colombo, Fremantle, Melbourne and Sydney. It must have been a good deal more relaxing than the similar voyage Lawrence had undertaken as a Medical Officer on HM Troopship *Miltiades* 37 years earlier through seas patrolled by U-boats.

They took two cabins to allow Lawrence to use one as a study. Throughout his life, he maintained well-defined compartments; he never entered a social arena unless his exit was clear. He was in the habit of carrying a collection of ruled index cards so if he could not physically escape, he could do some legitimate jottings on whatever was his current project.

On 28 January when they were nearing Port Said, Lawrence wrote a rather unenthusiastic letter to his secretary Lilian Pearce reporting that ship life with its 1000-plus passengers was quite uneventful on calm, grey, sunless seas. He reported that he and Anna both had a mild dose of flu and he was glad to have 'a quiet cabin as a sanctuary in this otherwise noisy ship'. He said there was 'too much food, a few interesting people among many dull, cinemas and dancing, deck games and gambling'. He ended unconvincingly with, 'Will join in some soon.' The crew on these long-distance voyages made every effort to fill the day with organized entertainment, and he was clearly glad to escape this. Anna always enjoyed meeting people and relaxing on board. She avoided flying whenever possible.

The programme in Australasia was organized by Dr Ewen Downie (1902–77), the physician in charge of the diabetic clinic at the Alfred Hospital, Melbourne, from 1929 to 1962 and the leading figure in the development of endocrinology as a subspecialty in Australia. He had been the official medical delegate for Australia at the inaugural IDF Congress in Leiden in 1952, which is where he had met Lawrence. The schedule included visits to Sydney, Brisbane, Melbourne, Adelaide and Perth, as well as a fishing holiday in New Zealand and a weekend in Tasmania. The inaugural meeting of the Victorian Diabetic Association was held in Melbourne on 24 March and Lawrence had been interviewed by Australian 3AW radio earlier in the day.

Anna reported to Lilian:

Moving around as often as we do it is not easy to settle down to writing to anyone except the family but today is quite free for me while Robin does a round of hospitals, clinics, lectures etc. Last night [24 March] was the inaugural meeting of the Victoria Diabetic Association. The press and media had given it a big build up; Robin had been interviewed and made recordings, etc.[1] and the result was the same as the Sydney Diabetic Association meeting: hall packed to suffocation and about 300 unable to get in. It seems unfortunate that they could not have hired larger halls; Sydney held 600: last night more than 700 squeezed in but such a crowd had not been anticipated. Anyhow it was all a great success, and members enrolled feverishly. Robin is not too tired, and the two trips to the fishing in NZ and Tasmania have been wonderful breaks. I'm enjoying it all, needless to say, and we seem to be getting on well with everybody. We would very much like to have gone inland to see the real Australia and a sheep station but there hasn't been the time.

Dr Hal Breidahl, who later worked in Lawrence's clinic in 1954–56, recalls an episode during one of the meetings:

When a photographer crept up to the table behind which Lawrence was speaking, he leant across, grabbed the man by his lapels, and said: 'Pay your subscription now – or no photograph.' The photographer was taken aback and paid up meekly.

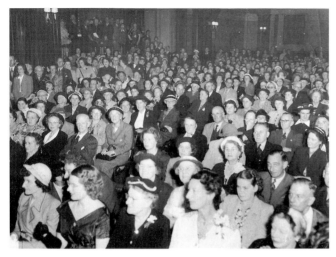

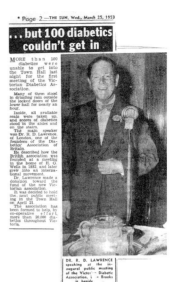

* Page 2 —THE SUN, Wed., March 25, 1953

.. but 100 diabetics couldn't get in

MORE than 100 diabetics were unable to get into the Town Hall last night for the first meeting of the Victorian Diabetics Association.

Many of them stood in drizzling rain outside the locked doors of the lower hall for nearly an hour.

Inside, all available seats were taken up, and scores of diabetics stood in the aisles and on the stairs.

The main speaker was Dr. R. D. Lawrence, of London, one of the founders of the Diabetics' Association of Britain.

He described how the British association was founded at a meeting in the home of H. G. Wells in 1933, and later grew into an international movement.

Dr. Lawrence made a donation toward the fund of the new Victorian association.

It was decided to hold the next public meeting in the Town Hall on April 21.

The association has been formed to help, by co-operative effort, more than 20,000 diabetics throughout Victoria.

DR. R. D. LAWRENCE speaking at the inaugural public meeting of the Victor' ~ Diabetic Association. L v Brooks is beside

Packed auditorium at the inaugural meeting of the Sydney Diabetic Association, March 1953.

Lawrence used a relaxed, conversational style for his lectures, with a favourite opening:

> I should really call you fellow diabetics because that is what I am. I suppose I have had diabetes longer than anyone else in the room – 33 years. Can anyone beat that?

His thunder was stolen by a hand that rose up: 'Right', said Lawrence: 'I will see you afterwards.'

Lawrence continued by outlining the foundation of the British Diabetic Association, and went on to describe some of the early activities:

> In the old days there was no free insulin in England, and there were people who could not afford enough food and we, personally, helped them and others with their economic difficulties and trials. And then there were the diabetic children. And there were no convalescent homes. If you sent a diabetic patient to a home you knew everything would go wrong. They were filled up with rice puddings, custards covered with sugar, and nothing else and often the insulin was not properly measured. So we managed to establish, among other things, a convalescent home for diabetics.[2] And that worked all right. We started them with our money but the Government then took over. We did not perpetually have to keep them going; we would have been completely ruined otherwise.
>
> We had holiday camps for diabetic children, who can be, even with the most loving and careful parents. a great tie; but if we can give the children two or three weeks' holiday in a summer camp we can in some way let the parents have a free time from the responsibility of their diabetic children.

He described the setting up of children's hostels:

> *There are always some diabetic children who, through no fault of their own, through careless or ignorant parents, are never looked after properly and spend most of their time in hospital in coma of one form or another – too much insulin or sometimes too little. Homes were established for them by the association and they are now paid for by the Minister of Education and 125 children are being brought up permanently in this way.*

He also reported the purchase of the old people's home:[3]

> *for old people who have not got families and cannot look after themselves. They are paid for by the local authorities and we do not have to maintain them.*
>
> *The greatest thing we have done is to start new movements and get them paid for by other people. You cannot really look after huge commitments without being ruined unless there are a few millionaires. Are there any millionaires sitting in the hall?*

Not one hand went up in response to this question.

Lawrence went on to talk about the formation of the IDF:

> *Fundamentally, diabetics everywhere have the same difficulties and problems in common, much worse in some countries. No free insulin, which is a terrible thing. They met last year, in two sections. One for the laymen to discuss their difficulties: in some countries, difficulties of employment, and prejudices against employment of diabetics. I do not blame entirely the employers because of the difficulties of superannuation and so on. This is the social side which the laymen handle. And then there is the more important side in which doctors and scientists are most interested – medical research which has kept most of you alive: certainly me. It is not a perfect treatment; it is not a bad life; but there can be a better one, and that will only arise from increase of knowledge, difficult work in the laboratory and that is the side of it we think is very important, not merely to keep you fit and well and normal as at present, but to make things better and that can only be achieved by the increase of knowledge. This is occurring very fast. In England diabetics themselves supply five thousand pounds a year for research. More is required everywhere. Research is not easy. To find out anything new and get down to the hidden mysteries of human diseases takes intricate and expensive equipment and prolonged study.*
>
> *That is what we have done and that is what I hope you will do. I think it would be a jolly nice idea if I started a subscription and became the first honorary member. I have talked long enough, perhaps too long, but I would just like to finish by saying that it is only two months ago, just before I left England, that Her Majesty the Queen became Patron of the Diabetic Association.*

And amid appreciative applause, Lawrence handed over his £1. According to J. G. L. Jackson it was 'a typical, barnstorming speech by RDL: brisk and succinct, and his audiences loved it'. There were many questions that he answered in the same direct way. One of them was from:

> a rather inebriated fellow, who rose and asked 'when are you going to get us some tablets instead of this damned insulin stuff?'

Lawrence's reply was moderate:

> No such preparation has yet been evolved

and then as Hal Breidhal recalled, 'in three years' time we had the sulphonylureas.'

From Melbourne, they went on to Adelaide, and later to Perth, from where Lawrence wrote to Lilian Pearce on Easter Sunday 5 April 1953:

> Here Bruce Hunt[4] vastly in charge but some leisure also. Glad to hear of almonds ~ flowering; here autumn, plenty of flowers but no blooming trees. Now to work answers:
> 1) back Thursday 9th (time unknown) and I presume Friday is devoted to letter problems only and we shall go and see Dan, Hayling and perhaps the farm Sat and Sunday: patients Monday usual time & KCH as usual.
> 2) Oh dear, this Hull business! No lecture to GPs. Certainly the meeting. Can I fly later than 9 am train? Anna will come up and we both go to see Adam, however briefly at Catterick Sat and Sunday and me back for usual work. I don't look forward to Hull, but will do what I must. Are you or many of the Council going?
> 3) please try the MRC for one possibly two Coronation tickets or anywhere else at about the same price of £6+.
> 4) I am not raising the Whittington article here but have done a lot about diabetic entrance to Australia.
> 5) I've raised much enthusiasm about Diabetic Associations in different states. Here much sun but quite cold winds morning and evening. A keen and interested medical profession everywhere, but I'm not learning much.

To this letter Anna added a note about the Coronation tickets, since Lawrence had obviously forgotten that she had already been in touch with Dan about them:

> It would be best I think if you and he communicated about this. The fact is that I would very much like to see it and not just televise it. I think Dan will be home – I don't know about Adam – but I'm sure Dan would like to see it, in real life, too, and what about you? It may be too late to get seats but I've been told by several Aussies that they have been offered them from several different sources and I imagine there may be some going at the last minute so to speak. (80,000 have been allotted Australia). The part of the route within walking distance of 8 Devonshire Place would obviously be the best. If you would like to come with us, please be our guest.

> Anna L.

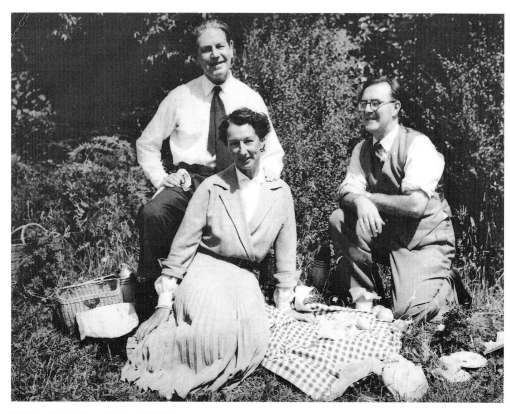

Fishing trip in New Zealand, 1953.

The Lawrences came home by sea on the P&O liner *Himalaya*: Anna was initiated as a Daughter of Neptune when crossing the Equator. On 29 April, they were in Port Said, when Lawrence scribbled a brief note to Lilian Pearce:

Last letter and back sometime as yet unknown on 7th. Book more or less finished and weather cooling almost too much. Mail not in yet but I shall post this before going ashore. So see you soon, Yours RDL.

Three years after the visit to Melbourne for the formation of the Diabetic Association in the state of Victoria, Ewen Downie wrote to Lawrence with a progress report:

Over 1100 members and a substantial credit balance show evidence of a strong and thriving organisation.

He went on to tell Lawrence that the formation of an Australian Diabetic Association was well underway. In fact, the inaugural meeting of the Diabetes Federation of Australia was held in Sydney in October 1957.

According to Jackson, the reference to 'this Hull business' in Lawrence's letter of 5 April concerned the AGM of the British Diabetic Association, which for the first time was to be held outside London. Hull had been selected owing to pressure exerted by the forceful representative of the Branch, Councillor Alderman R. E. Smith, and Lawrence was not at all enthusiastic about the idea. In the event, it was a considerable success. After an informal tea, a coach trip was organized to Trinity House, and this was followed by a civic reception and dinner in the Guildhall, arranged by the Lord Mayor of Hull, who was himself a diabetic. Some 400 members assembled in the Guildhall for the AGM, which was chaired by Lord Hotham, a Vice-President of the BDA, in the unavoidable absence of Mr Henriques, the President. Lawrence gave one of his usual enthusiastic talks and Jackson recorded that it was 'greatly appreciated'.

In 1954 Charles Best had a heart attack. Lawrence wrote:

My dear Charley and all, but particularly Charley because I want to know about health and future movements and travellings. I have joyed to gather from various sources that you are near A1 again. I pray, unusual for me, for this … Now to business.

1. *You are come to Ciba symposium.*
2. *The IDF at Cambridge too. Do you want a hotel room for you and Margaret or do you stay with friends? Congress arrangements in good order. Lionel Whitby [Regius Professor of Physic at Cambridge] to be Honorary President; the Senate House for 1st ceremony. Dear Joslin is going to give the Banting Memorial Lecture. I hope to get Ciba scientists to give a few papers. Can you suggest who might be the best and would the real Best think of a paper himself? And you'll let us know anything on earth we can do for all of you in England – money, a car etc. etc.*
3. *And, v confidentially, there are shocking tensions in the IDF Exec Board between the French Paz and Fritz G[erritzen], the clashing of v dissimilar temperaments. Poor me has had to intervene in this threatening situation. I am a man of peace and compromise and there is none of the latter in Paz.*
4. *Now to better things … I am to give the Lilley Lecture at the American College Physicians' meeting, Philadelphia end April 1955. Anna coming and her expenses paid too. Good old Eli! I doubt if we shall even attempt to visit you in Toronto then on a short visit. But, by Jove, we'll hear your voices by phone.*
5. *Family news. Ours all well but seldom at home and Anna loves a full house. Rob (24) working intelligently at St. Thomas' but with growing cultural interest: Adam (21) – Cambridge Anatomy (too much) and Physg. Dan (18) trying for a place at Oxford before his horrible military 2 years service. None enormously clever academically, but good characters and citizens. I know your boys combine both these virtues.*
   Enough to make I hope yours and my most friendly contact for ever. And now to four more clinical diabetic problems. Blessings, Robin L and Anna too. Miss ye all –

Section 5 of this letter gives a glimpse into the high standards by which Lawrence judged his sons. Rob was working as a doctor, Adam at Cambridge studying medicine and playing Real Tennis for the University, and Dan aiming for

Oxford entry (he eventually went to Cambridge), yet Lawrence downplays their achievements and abilities.

As indicated in his letter to Best, Lawrence was honoured by an invitation to deliver the 1955 Lilly Lecture of the American Diabetes Association, and he travelled there with Anna in April. Writing to Lilian Pearce on 1 May, from Atlantic City, he said:

> *All going well, but here our first leisure. A super Brighton, but not much good weather. Lilly Lecture went well. RDL*

To this card, Anna added:

> *Indeed it did. Life here less hectically organised and some time to take in the sun. Sea freezing. Best wishes, AL.*

By 17 May, they were in New York, staying at The Tuscany Hotel:

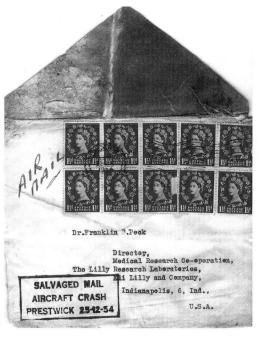

Lawrence corresponded with The Lilly Laboratories before his US trip. This letter with Lilian Pearce's handwritten 'Air Mail' was returned to him after it was salvaged from the plane crash at Prestwick that killed 28 of the 36 passengers on board.

Embarking tomorrow and I know I haven't written a single letter to anyone at home and only a few thanking Americans for their hospitality. Too bad! The whole tour has been such a filled-up rush that the pen has been neglected. I lunched with Connolly[5] and heard the good news that he is coming to Cambridge. I've met hundreds of doctors and some are wondering about the date of their papers at IDF. That must be the first job on return. You've probably got it all in order.

The Second IDF Congress in Cambridge in 1955 attracted 500 participants from 30 countries and was blessed with fine weather. Lawrence and Anna stayed in the Garden House Hotel, along with Charles Best and Margaret, Elliot Joslin, with his son Allen and family, Dr and Mrs Fritz Gerritzen, Mr Pieter Duys, and others. After the opening ceremony in the Senate House of the University, Joslin gave the Ninth Banting Memorial Lecture of the British Diabetic Association to a crowded hall. Another highlight of that week was the dinner given in Trinity Hall (organized by Adam Lawrence who was a student there at the time) by the Executive Council of the BDA to the official delegates from other member associations of the IDF: 55 representatives of 18 countries. The chair was taken by Sir Basil Henriques, the newly knighted President of the BDA, and speeches were made by him, by Dr Howard Root (United States), Dr F. F. (Francisco) Rocca (Uruguay), Dr A. Hey

(Denmark), Dr H. J. Banse (Germany), Mr J. P. McNulty (Ireland) and Mlle J. M. Piguet (France). Rather surprisingly, Lawrence did not make a speech, perhaps because he was preoccupied with the problem of what to do about Maurice Paz, President of the predominantly lay French association, who wanted the IDF to be more active in promoting the social needs of the diabetic community. When the medically dominated Executive Council refused to accede to his demands, Paz resigned as a Vice-President of IDF, but then withdrew his resignation, and continued his campaign through the French journal in a series of articles, extremely critical of the Dutch Secretariat. These continued throughout the next two years, during which time Gerritzen and Pieter Duys struggled to maintain the momentum they had created from the Dutch headquarters. But eventually, Duys, owing to family and personal illness, was unable to carry on, and Gerritzen also submitted his resignation. The Executive Board of the IDF met in Brussels in July 1956, when Paz, on vacation, was unable to attend.

The possibility of moving the headquarters of IDF to Geneva, where it might 'be blessed financially by WHO' was found to be impossible, following enquiries by Professor Rambert, of Paris, and others. Without such support, the income from IDF Member Associations was far too small to support such a scheme. It was therefore decided to move the headquarters to London, in a room rented from the BDA, but quite independent from them. Lawrence was able to engage the services of Dr L. L. Frank, an American living in London, who was a Fellow of the American Diabetes Association and of the American College of Physicians, to act as Secretary, with Mr David Brown, FCA, a patient of Lawrence and a member of the Council of the BDA, as Treasurer. The *IDF News Bulletin* of January 1957 carried a leading article by Lawrence outlining the reasons for the changes, and paying tribute to the pioneer work of Dr Gerritzen and Mr Duys. As far as Maurice Paz was concerned:

> *The Executive Board also considered the perpetually critical attitude of M. Paz of the IDF Secretariat and the IDF as published for years in the French journal over his name. It was unanimously felt by vote that his attitude was detrimental to the relations of France to the IDF and it has been suggested to him that he should resign again, as he did at Cambridge in 1955. Personal antagonisms and quarrels are to me impossible to understand in an association devoted to the welfare of diabetics all over the world.*

The extreme shortage of funds prevented the IDF from expanding its activities:

> *as you and I would like ... I hope that the changes we have had to make may conserve and expand the life and activities of the IDF. The changes have been partly caused by personal tensions, most distressing to me in a movement devoted to the help of diabetics all over the world.*

These problems gave Lawrence a great deal of concern, in part owing to his loyalty to Gerritzen and Hoet, old friends, whose families he knew well, and whose sons had studied under Charles Best in Toronto along with his own eldest son, Rob. His natural instinct was to ignore such matters and hope they would go away, but he was forced to take action, and did so decisively.

Professor Rolf Luft (1914–2007), who was President of the IDF from 1973 to 1980, recalls his first meeting with Lawrence, at Cambridge:

> *I had heard of him but his appearance surpassed my expectations: this figure in striped trousers, morning-coat and a red carnation appeared to me like a joke. In addition, he seemed to me pompous and dominating without any scientific basis for his statements. Let me say that I did not, at this time, appreciate his great qualities.*
>
> *The next time was around 1958, when I gave a lecture to the BDA on hypophysectomy[6] in diabetics with advanced retinopathy. I think it was at the Royal Society of Medicine. When I entered a reception, I saw Lawrence in the middle of the room keeping court, surrounded by a substantial group of people. I approached, he saw me, turned round and said, 'Sir, are you the one who removes the hypophysis in diabetic patients?' I said, 'Yes, Dr Lawrence.' 'How dare you, sir; how dare you!' Then I caught fire. I explained to him that I cared for the patients as much as he did, but I did not wish to watch one after the other going blind. I also emphasised that I did not consider hypophysectomy the ultimate therapy, but that this approach had opened the road to novel attempts to stop the complications, i.e. by medical means to stop the production of pituitary growth hormone. He grumbled something like: 'I hope so, good luck' or something similar, turned his back on me, and continued to talk to the people around him. At this moment I understood him better, and I sort of liked his attack on me. He stood up for the patients; he wasn't scared by such a bold endeavour. And he was a diabetic himself and identified with the patients. I looked upon him with new eyes. He was a caring physician, a little strange to me but not pompous.*

Luft later recalled of Lawrence that:

> *He was interesting to talk to. In essence, he was satisfied with the care he had given his patients but was fully aware of the negative side. My message was that doctors like him, Joslin, Hoet and others had contributed a lot to the development of diabetes care but that, in the future, this type of care delivered by knowledgeable patriarchal persons could never reach the diabetic community but only isolated patients. He agreed. It was a nice talk with a real gentleman and warm-hearted humorous person.*

South Africa's application for membership of the IDF caused concern. Lawrence felt strongly that there were gross discrepancies in the remuneration of white and coloured doctors, as they were called at the time, which in his view was an offence against the accepted principles of medical ethics, and was totally opposed to the BDA sponsoring the South African Society. Opposing views were put forward by other Council members, who felt that the question of colour discrimination in South Africa was irrelevant: what mattered was whether the admission of the Society would work for the benefit of the IDF. By vote, the Council agreed to sponsor the application, by 11 to 1, Lawrence being the only opposer, although there were 4 abstentions. The difficulty of obtaining an additional sponsor for South Africa meant that their application was not processed until 1964, when the Council approved the admission without dissent.

The IDF continues to grow in stature and importance. Today, it is an umbrella organization of over 200 national diabetes associations in over 160 countries acting to tackle diabetes at local or international level with educational programmes, support for national and international policies on diabetes, and research grants. A world congress is held every two years, attracting up to 12,000 international delegates. The IDF is part of the World Health Organization's global, non-communicable disease network and assists in collecting data to show how common diabetes is in different countries and its increasing prevalence. The IDF helped to achieve a UN resolution on diabetes in 2006 and World Diabetes Day is an official UN World Day.

Towards the end of 1963, there were discussions within Europe about a new diabetes journal. Lawrence sought the views of his colleagues at King's College Hospital, all of whom felt that (in Lawrence's words):

as 'Diabetes' (the journal of the American Diabetes Association) is going to be published monthly in the near future, there is probably no need for a European Journal. In any case, the success of such a journal must have a minimum guaranteed subscription. An Editorial Board must be set up. Much more information is required.

To this note in his files is added what are probably the comments of Lilian Pearce:

It may be that some of the European countries, i.e. Germany and some of the smaller countries (say Holland, Belgium) would be in favour of this production because:
a) *it would no doubt be published in three languages – English, German and French.*
b) *it may be difficult for these countries to get articles published in the American 'Diabetes'.*
c) *Professor Renold (ex USA) now working in Switzerland is in favour of this project; it is thought mainly because it would give him – as well as others – an outlet for publications.*

Against this final sentence, Lawrence has written 'perhaps poor' – which might be taken as a somewhat autocratic disinclination to recognize the growth of good European research.

A founding group of diabetologists came together at the Fifth International meeting of the IDF in 1964, and the first meeting of the newly formed European Association for the Study of Diabetes (EASD) took place in April 1965 at Montecatini in Italy, and the new journal, *Diabetologia*, was launched in August 1965 as a quarterly. Despite his concerns, Lawrence was elected as an Honorary Member.

References

1. This interview can be heard in full at http://www.diabetes-stories.com/index.asp

2. Burley on the Hill, Rutland, in 1946.
3. Frederick Banting House on Kingston Hill was ready for opening in 1954.
4. Bruce Hunt (1899–1964) was a controversial character who believed in free diets for diabetics.
5. J. Richard Connolly (1917–77) was Executive Director of the American Diabetes Association.
6. Hypophysectomy is the surgical removal of the pituitary gland (hypophysis).

CHAPTER 11

Patients and Colleagues

The wisdom and compassion he bestowed on me has enriched and protected my life

Beatrice Reid, patient of Lawrence, on insulin for 70 years

In 1953, Lawrence gave a talk on Australian Radio to 'the diabetics of Australia' who he called 'fellow diabetics' saying he was one himself and had been for a third of a century. He was looking forward to reaching 50 before being 'bowled out'. He went on to say that it was because diabetes took him up that he took up the study of it as his life work. He viewed this as a great advantage as, 'it brings more intimate knowledge, understanding and sympathy, I hope, to my patients.'

Lawrence was an astute clinician who knew his patients well. In an obituary Christopher Hardwick, physician in charge of the diabetic clinic at Guy's wrote that:

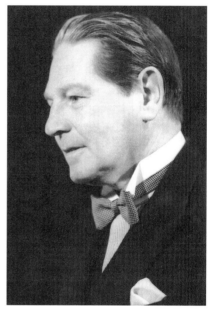

RD Lawrence.

> [in a very busy clinic] Lawrence himself did more than his share of the work, for not only did he teach the students, but often there would be distinguished visitors from abroad as well. These visitors learned much about the management of diabetes, but they also had an outstanding lesson in the care of patients, for Lawrence seemed to know them all by name and he appeared to be acquainted with the personal problems of most of them.[1]

When Jim Jackson was preparing material for Lawrence's biography, he put a request in *Balance* in 1989 for recollections from former patients and colleagues. Although Lawrence had died 21 years earlier, nearly 50 letters were received. All mentioned his knowledge, understanding and sympathy. Many remembered their first visit to Lawrence as children. One was from a woman who had lived with diabetes for 63 years and had seen Lawrence regularly over 32 years since her diagnosis in 1926. She especially welcomed the changes in the diet over the years. She remembered her mother putting bran in a muslin bag which was tied to the cold water tap for 24 hours until it ran clear. The bran was then mixed with agar and baked to form what must have been a very dry biscuit. She finished by saying her only wish was that dear Dr Lawrence was here today to see how much progress has been made in diet and in the management of the disease.

Lawrence made a strong and lasting impression on the children he treated. Many were initially overawed by his formal attire, and all mentioned the carnation buttonhole. In all these letters there was a strong sense of pride that such a smart doctor should be interested in them, a mere child. However autocratic his manner might have been towards some colleagues, he was sympathetic and insightful with the children. He never patronized them and they were quick to appreciate this.

Many were touched by the way the great doctor knelt down to be at the child's level. He took them into his confidence, speaking directly to them rather than over their heads to the parent. Several writers noted how comforting it was to know that this grand-looking doctor was also diabetic and had to endure needles, blood and urine tests and various dietary restrictions, just like the children.

One young patient had an appointment on her 15th birthday and was touched that Lawrence remembered to wish her many happy returns. On one appointment there were several other people waiting to see him and the girl's mother remarked: 'You are very busy this morning, Dr. Lawrence.' His reply was: 'Well, you see the bounders all live now'. She recalled that this remark was typical of his droll sense of humour which was one of the things for which she would always remember him. Like many patients, she found *The Diabetic Life* a constant source of reassurance and comfort that was a tangible reminder of a remarkable man whom she would always regard with the utmost affection. Over and again, patients stated how *The Diabetic Life* became their bible.

Patients appreciated his blunt, unequivocal approach. One young woman became depressed with having to inject herself, so her mother took her to a dietetic clinic, where she was given a diet to follow with plenty of meat and fruit. She continued on this diet for some time, not having any insulin, or testing her urine. She began to lose weight and suffer with boils, and was sent to Kings, where she remembered Lawrence saying, 'You either go back on to insulin, or you will not be here in a year's time'.

A revealing portrait of Lawrence, and of the treatment of diabetes away from the main centres, came from a letter by a woman who wrote:

I was diagnosed diabetic, after just one term at infant school, during the Christmas holiday of 1940, when many people, including my mother, whose brother had died from it, aged eleven in 1914, still thought it meant certain death to a child. After a visit to our GP and having been assured that I was not going to die, we were sent to see the physician at our local hospital, who, before my parents could explain and reassure me, had me whisked away to the children's' ward, where I spent six weeks of fear and much unhappiness, thinking that this thing the doctor said I'd got was something I must have done which was so bad that my parents didn't want me any more. This experience, and the heartless way we were treated on the ward, left me, for many years, with a dread of hospitals. I came home at last, feeling like a leper, to a very strict diet of high protein and very low carbohydrate, two injections a day and the awful news that if I ever ate a sweet, cake or biscuit again, I would die a slow and painful death.

Her father, a schoolmaster was horrified by what he considered an absurd diet for a five year old and saved up for a year to take her to see Lawrence in Bath. She continued:

After introducing himself to each of us in turn, he spoke to my parents for a few minutes, then turned to me, and, taking hold of my hands, he crouched down to my height, telling me that he'd heard that I'd been a very good girl, that I'd not made a fuss about having injections and that it must have been very boring for me to have to eat the same things each day, and that he would have been bored too. Then, still holding my hand, he led me to a chair, asked me to sit on it, and explained that he was going to prick my ear, take a drop of blood from it and test it; that it would only be a little prick and that he knew that someone who had two injections every day would be just as brave about this.

He explained that he was going to put me on a different sort of diet, when I could eat lots of different things, and not only that, but that he was going to change my injections to one a day, to be done each morning before breakfast, just as my first one was, but that this injection would have two insulins in it that meant it would last till the next day, and that he expected that it would be nicer for me; but that it was almost certain that I would have to have an injection every day for the rest of my life, but that I would get so used to it that it wouldn't matter to me after a bit: also that I would always have to be careful about what I ate, but that as I grew older, and learnt more about it, I would be able to do all the things that my friends did.

Then he turned to my parents and said: 'Don't exclude all treats from her; let her have a few sweets or chocolate' (I could hardly believe my ears) 'a square of milk chocolate or a boiled sweet is about five grams of carbohydrate, and as long as she is well and stable it will do her no harm to have them, as long as you make them part of her allowance for tea or instead of her last 10 grams before bed.' And having added some advice about parties, he turned back to me and said: 'I know that you will be a sensible girl, and am sure you can be trusted not to eat things you know you shouldn't eat when away from home, but sometimes, however hard you try not to do something, we find it too hard to say "no", and I want you to promise me that if you ever do eat sweets or cake or anything you know you shouldn't have, you will tell your mother that you have and how much, so that she can make sure that it doesn't make you poorly, and I promise you that if you do this, and you really have tried not to, but just couldn't help it, she won't be cross with you; but it really is best not to if you can manage it.'

A parent whose toddler was diagnosed at King's when 20 months old remembered how much the child had enjoyed the children's Christmas parties at the hospital where Lawrence played the part of Father Christmas. For the rest of the year, she particularly valued Lawrence's formal attire which gave him a distinctive and dignified appearance.

One patient wrote:

I remember, as a rebellious seven year old, kicking against injections and food rules, how Dr. Lawrence took the wind out of my sails by telling me I could eat whatever I liked; all I had to do was to remember what I had eaten and tell my mum about it, and not try to deceive her or myself. It did not take me long to put this teaching into practice. At school, my teacher and my classmates knew about my diabetes and that I had to eat one large banana, twenty grams carbohydrate, at break. This routine bored me stiff. I cut my banana in two, ten grams each, and started to swap with what my class friends had brought for their mid-morning break. Banana was a novelty for them and they were as keen to try it as I was to be rid of it. This developed into a fascinating barter system. One day half a banana was swapped for a digestive biscuit, next day for half a sandwich, then for three toffees. Becoming braver, both halves of the banana were exchanged for a biscuit and an apple, or an orange and ten Smarties. Break became exciting, not boring. I did not feel deprived any longer and have not done so since. I remembered the second part of Dr. Lawrence's instructions. I always told my mother exactly what I had eaten and I was always praised for doing this. When she called to collect me from school, my friends would rush over to tell her all about that day's banana exchanges!

One of Lawrence's most remarkable patients was Beatrice Reid, who was on insulin for over 70 years and embraced all Lawrence's commonsense principles wholeheartedly. He emphasized the need to avoid invalidism and she adopted this approach with commendable enthusiasm by stating robustly:

Diabetes is not an illness any more than having red hair or flat feet is an illness. It is a permanent condition that has to be accepted and organized. If anyone from the diabetic establishment tries to persuade you that you have an illness, close your ears and go elsewhere for help and guidance.

She particularly appreciated the way he was a partner working together to establish the patient's health. She recalled one of her childhood visits to him:

After a friendly exchange of family news, I remember he would always ask to be shown the glucose sweets I was carrying. He would explain, with a twinkle in his eye, that in the past his patients had seemed too good to be true. Every one of them said they always carried glucose sweets ready for an emergency. When he asked to see what they were carrying, he found his fears were justified. Only about one in ten could produce the sweets they said they had. He told me he wouldn't like me to be one of those irresponsible people who go around without the sugar they will need to counteract a hypo.

The next conversation would be about blood sugar. Dr. Lawrence would say,

'We'll both guess what we think your blood sugar is now. I'll write down the answers and put them in front of us on my desk. No cheating! Of course, you should be right and I should be wrong. I can't expect to know as much about how your body works as you can.' Sometimes we were both slightly wrong but most times I was the winner.

We would then discuss the new medium and long-lasting insulins that were coming on to the market. He would try them out on himself in different strengths and combinations. He would often say, 'Your diabetes seems to be happy as it is. I see no advantage for you in disturbing things. Why should you change?' This seems to be an excellent way of empowering the child patient.

She always remembered the message Dr. Lawrence passed on to her:

Never let diabetes stop you doing anything you want to do. And remember you must control your diabetes: never let it control you.

A mother whose son had developed diabetes timidly suggested to Lawrence that a parent practise giving an injection into an orange or a grapefruit rather than experiment on their child:

Dr. Lawrence looked across at me with the most piercing gaze, 'do you know?' he said, 'That's a thunderingly good idea' and he started writing it in his notebook.

The parent really appreciated the way her idea had been taken up. When the family went out to Australia, Lawrence wrote a letter to a colleague in Sydney who later read aloud part of the referral letter to the boy's mother, 'J has the most priceless of gifts, a highly intelligent mother.'

The experience of children was less pleasant if they were not private patients. One remembered being admitted to King's with newly diagnosed diabetes in 1932 when she was 10. In the children's ward, as was common at the time, visiting was only allowed on Sundays, but her mother came every evening to leave a parcel of goodies and toys. She stayed in hospital for three weeks and every day was given lessons in diet. At discharge, her parents had to buy all the equipment, such as syringes, syringe cases and scales for weighing the food – she remembers that bottle of 40 units/cm^3 insulin cost 4 shillings. At first, she attended the clinic, which excitingly for a child was held upstairs in the pathology laboratory, every three weeks:

The waiting room was very small, and if a dozen patients attended it was a crowd, for there were only about 200 diabetic patients on the books ... over the years the number of patients attending the clinic increased. We often had very long waits and were obliged to listen to very gruesome tales from some of the adults.

During 1962, Lawrence was touched to receive the following letter from one of his patients, who wrote because he had recently met Lawrence's son, Adam, at St. Thomas's Hospital:

I must truly record to you how impressed I was with his gentleness and kindness.

and then added:

I felt I must say to you how humbly grateful I am to you for enabling me to live with my diabetes for the past 22 years. In the past, I haven't been a model patient. I'm not sure that I'm as good as I ought to be even now – though I've reformed a great deal over the last two years or so. But somehow I don't think that I would have lasted the course this far without your very highly personalised treatment – which has gone far beyond prescribing insulin, even to include education and assistance in finding a personal philosophy of Life that allows for diabetes without diabetes becoming an excuse for indulgence and self-pity. All of which is to say that, inevitably, I have met and talked to other diabetics and heard of the treatment in their particular cases from other doctors. And that particular brand of treatment wouldn't have preserved me for over two decades.

So for Life, for enabling me to marry, for my family, for fun, for my ability to enjoy music and plays and films and, particularly, books; for all the pleasure I derive from my garden and its plants and the trees and birds and fields, for country walks and dinners in town with good wine and good company – oh, the list is endless, but absolutely most of all for the love of my small sons – thank you, Dr. Lawrence. Thank you, very, very, much.

One mother wrote to thank him for looking after her daughter:

Over the past ten years you have educated my daughter to be as independent and happy a person as one could ever hope.

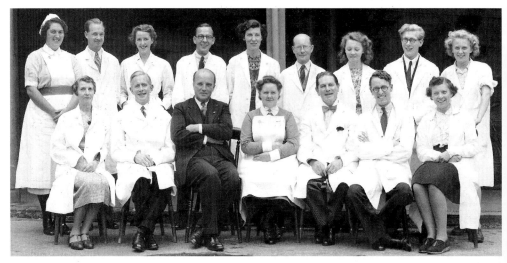

Colleagues at King's College Hospital. Charles Best (in suit) visit to KCH to celebrate 25th anniversary of the discovery of insulin.

Another patient wrote that there were no adequate words to say:

thank you for a life changed from weakness and weariness to strength and happiness.

Lawrence's colleagues also responded to the request by Jackson for memories. Dr. Phyllis Edwards (1911–2003) who qualified at King's in 1935 wrote:[2]

Dr. Lawrence always arrived for his outpatient clinics on time and fastidiously dressed, often with a flower in his buttonhole. His courtesy to the poorest of his patients – and many in those days were terribly poor, and his patience in explaining the treatment they were to undergo were in sharp contrast to the brusque manners and dismissive commands other consultants whose clinics and ward rounds I had attended as a student. He was a keen squash player and if an odd half hour of leisure could be snatched he loved a really hard game, which meant that, he would need to take some extra carbohydrate so he always carried a bar of chocolate in readiness and always gave a half of it to his house physician.

A doctor who was his Medical Registrar for three years in the late 1940s wrote that:

He was a great teacher and a delightful man to work for. Lawrence did not always follow what he preached: he told me that in order to enjoy some meal at a restaurant or a dinner to which he was invited he would look at the menu and assess what he would require in the way of extra insulin to cope with it and would then inject himself through his trousers under the table and then eat and drink what he fancied: in order to do this however you need to know what you are about – as he did.

Another wrote:

During the war, our MO went into the RAF. We had a locum from London. I told him I would not be on duty the following day as I had an appointment to see Dr. Lawrence at Harley Street. The locum said that whilst he was working in town he was called to a police station to examine a Dr Lawrence who was thought to be under the influence: the locum diagnosed him to be hypoglycaemic.

Mr K. C. McKeown, later a distinguished surgeon in Darlington, credits Lawrence with being the first to distinguish between arteriosclerotic and neurogenic gangrene in the diabetic foot.[1] When he was a junior surgeon at King's in 1941, the standard treatment for gangrene in the diabetic foot was an above knee amputation. This was done to avoid the problem of the stump not healing, as happened in older patients if the arteries in the leg were blocked.

He remembered that in 1941 Lawrence showed him a patient and said, 'I want you to amputate the foot partly.' He was horrified and protested that what he was being asked to do was completely unsurgical and bore no relation to any of the known techniques for amputations of the feet. What Lawrence was asking the young surgeon to do was a wedge resection of the foot, in McKeown's words, 'just like cutting a section out of a cake. He said he would take full responsibility and because of this I reluctantly agreed to do it.'

In fact, as Lawrence had realized, the blood supply to the foot was good because the so called 'gangrene' was caused by infection not hardening of the arteries. The wound was left open and, as McKeown remembered:

> *The foot healed so well that one did not realize that the toe was missing. The results of this procedure were quite excellent and I did many of them.*

McKeown worked closely with Lawrence until 1944, when he went into the Army. He recalls that when Lawrence became hypoglycaemic, he got very cross. McKeown wrote:

> *Because of this, he always had a lady House Physician to calm him down. When I played tennis with him he was excellent in the first set, but got rather wild in the second as he became hypoglycaemic. If you could persuade him to stop for tea, all would go well and his skills were restored. He was a man of strong likes and dislikes; fortunately we got on well.*

Lawrence appointed several women to his unit but had very traditional views about their role. This was exemplified in the case of Helen Jordan (later Pond) who became his house physician in December 1944. In 1989 she wrote to Jim Jackson that:

> *He struck me immediately as a kindly man; a 'big' man in the nicest possible way. Magnanimous, with a big brain and a large personality, slightly old-fashioned in a frock coat and a bit of showmanship with the red carnation in the button-hole. In those days we called our seniors 'Sir', and he never addressed me by my Christian name. We met them and saw them off at the door, and carried briefcases, etc. Hence I know that he was not very careful with his car: bumpers were definitely for bumping, and he rather barged! He only came to King's two days a week and was mostly in Harley Street. However, he always arrived 15–20 minutes before the clinic so that anyone of the staff could talk to him about personal or clinic matters without an appointment. Like all experienced physicians he was very good and quick with patients. He always knew at once what they needed in dosage and was almost always right. Perhaps he was too quick for some patients who wanted to talk. He was also sometimes impatient with students who wanted to know the reasoning behind his, often dramatic, treatment results. He did out-patients from 10 am–11.30 am by which time coffee and biscuits were urgently needed! He looked after his diabetes so well that he was frequently a little 'hypo'; House Physicians needed to know that his sugar lumps were in the left-hand waistcoat pocket! After coffee, he did a ward round until lunch.*

Helen was offered a research job, but there was trouble when Lawrence heard that she was engaged to be married. He took her out to lunch at Claridges to try to dissuade her and, when that failed, he took her and Desmond* out to dinner. Helen wrote:

> *That was not such a happy occasion. Lawrence thought Desmond a self-opinionated young man, and, what was worse, he couldn't dance! Lawrence was quite a good dancer by contrast. The frock-coat personality came to the fore over my marriage – either I would be a physician/research worker in diabetes, or I would be a married woman and leave my brain outside the door – both or a mixture. The only good mark Desmond got was that he was an exceptional musician, as was RDL, and they both loved Beethoven. He wrote me a charming note on my marriage, but five years later I was not acceptable to work with him again. I had transgressed and he stuck to his ideas about married women and their place in the home. However, I finally wore him down, and when his dear Katy Madders left in 1952, I was allowed to become an assistant in the out-patient department, dealing with diabetic children. I never had any paediatric qualifications, but Lawrence thought two children of my own would count as experience. I was very fond of him, and his teaching was influential.*

John A Hunt who was Lawrence's registrar in 1955 before emigrating to Canada, remembered that his boss refused to have anything to do with dieticians, maintaining that patients ate food, not calories. All teaching of diet was done by the ward cook and the two staff nurses, all of whom also ate food. This was not without its problems and Hunt remembered asking a patient what she had eaten the previous day:

> *The answer was: roast beef, Yorkshire pudding, roast potatoes and cabbage. I asked about the previous day, and got the same answer. And the previous day? Again, the same. So I asked why always the same? The answer was that that was the last meal that she had had in the diabetes ward; she couldn't remember any of the previous meals, so if she kept to it she would be sure not to make a mistake.*

Hunt remembered going to Lawrence's home for dinner and, unlike many juniors invited to dinner with the boss, felt very much at ease. He wrote:

> *Everything was totally relaxed, rather untidy, and extremely functional. One got the impression that he did all his reading in the living room at Devonshire Place with his desk in the corner by a window and things never quite got put away.*

Hunt also recalled the 'firm' dinner:

> *He had his insulin and syringe sitting on the table. A couple of times during the evening he grabbed them, drew up a dose of insulin, and injected himself straight through his trouser leg. He certainly did not believe in a restricted diabetic diet, or not for himself on social occasions. I think that he fostered in me an essentially*

---

* Desmond Pond (1919–1986). Later president of the Royal College of Psychiatrists and knighted.

practical approach to the management of diabetes, which has led me to encourage my patients to enjoy a highly varied life, choose an insulin schedule that seems appropriate, and then teach them to make adjustments to maintain the best possible control.

A young Australian physician, Hal Breidahl, met Lawrence in 1953 and was encouraged to come to London. Unfortunately, Hal did not realize until he came that no pay or living expenses were on offer. His assessment of Lawrence was that:

To some of his medical colleagues, he appeared arrogant and insufferable. He was undoubtedly dictatorial, and did not suffer fools gladly. He recognized talent, and knew how to bring the best out of those who worked for him. If he did not like someone, that person was never admitted to his social circle. But to those he liked, he was kind and thoughtful.

John Malins (1915–1992), whose diabetic clinic in Birmingham became almost as famous as the one at King's, knew Lawrence well. He remembered that:

When I first saw him I was struck by his handsome and attractive looks with a suggestion of Byronic wickedness, emphasized by his blind eye. His reputation was mixed. Some colleagues at King's regarded him as almost a charlatan, with no good reason, I suspect, and other physicians interested in diabetes were hostile, often from jealousy. George Graham of Bart's had been keen on diabetes at the right time but had no charisma. Lawrence had a huge practice and his patients adored him. He was very shrewd, understood their limitations and did not bully them. He was very kind to me and advised Birmingham patients who were referred to him to rely on me: that was not always easy. At diabetic meetings he assumed correctly that he was the Maestro and some did not enjoy that, but he was witty and his interjections were always to the point. I do not know much about his relations with the BDA, some thought he used it to his own advantage but it would have been difficult for him to avoid that.

Lawrence dominated the diabetic scene in Britain to a unique extent from the mid-1920s until the 1950s and it is not surprising that this, coupled with his flamboyant character led to jealousy and resentment among those outside his unit. Those who worked for him at King's in junior capacities seem to have been uniformly approving and admiring. Katie Madders (1884–1974) had worked closely with Lawrence during the early days at King's and wrote to him in 1952 saying how much affection she had for the Diabetic Clinic 'and above all for yourself.' She summed up by saying, 'The Clinic owes you not only its existence but its organization, enterprise, and its particularly human spirit.'

The person with whom there were tensions was Wilfrid Oakley. Oakley felt that Lawrence should have retired much earlier and was also affronted that he was not included in the Lawrence's social circle. Lawrence may well have felt that Oakley was less than fully committed to his NHS patients and more interested in Harley Street. Unfortunately we have no reliable information about what each thought about the other. Oakley later contributed Lawrence's entry for Munk's Roll [the lives of fellows of the Royal College of Physicians] which rather damned his colleague with faint praise. He wrote that:

> Both in his teaching and writing Lawrence aimed at simplicity of thought and expression; he sometimes underrated the intelligence of his audience. He was a most successful beggar in the cause of diabetes and a great believer in spending capital. Although an extrovert, some thought an exhibitionist, his scientific modesty made him unwilling to do more by way of correcting his juniors than to suggest a better alternative.

References

1. BMJ 1968; **3**: 621.
2. Review of The Diabetic Life 14th Edtition. *Postgrad Med J* 1950; **26**: 673.

CHAPTER 12

Doctor and Scientist: Lawrence's Clinical and Scientific Publications

Within two months of being diagnosed with diabetes in November 1920, Lawrence moved to the laboratory of Dr G. A. Harrison who, as we saw in Chapter 1, had already started studies on dietary treatment.[1] Now Lawrence himself turned to biochemical research on diabetes, at a time when he was slowly dying from the same disease. He studied levels of the pancreatic enzyme diastase (amylase) in blood and urine, concluding that they were of no value in the diagnosis, prognosis or treatment of diabetes. He was awarded his MD in March 1922, and the paper describing this research was published in February 1923,[2] just three months before he started insulin.

Remarkably, Lawrence's first 10 papers were published between 1924 and 1927, and included the results of self-experimentation. They provide an abundance of astute clinical observations, without doubt enhanced by his own experience, at a time when the use of insulin was scarcely understood. Later, he wrote that 'the twin sisters of clinical observation and laboratory experiment have walked, in the field of diabetes, very closely hand in hand'.[3] It was these 'twins' that he pursued for almost half a century and that are recorded in around 200 papers and case reports. His writing was a model of clarity and authority, and a pleasure to read.

Lawrence's earliest and crucial observations related to the concept that the amount of insulin had to be balanced by the carbohydrate intake. Throughout the 1920s, he examined both the necessary dietary requirements and the actions of insulin to enable his patients to

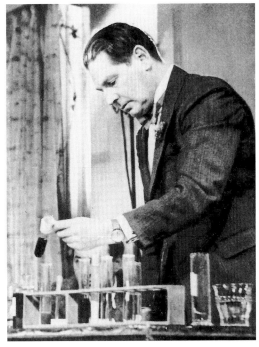

Lawrence on the BBC programme 'Matters of Life and Death', 1949.

manage their own condition. He introduced the line ration scheme for diabetic diets as early as 1924 (and published in 1925[4]), a scheme that stood the test of time over several decades. He believed that patients could grasp this programme 'in two minutes', and was easily understood by those who were 'not very intelligent'. With G. A. Harrison, he produced a booklet *Food Tables: Compiled Particularly for the Use in Treatment of Diabetes Mellitus*. The first edition was printed privately,[5] with a second edition being published in 1924.[6]

One of Lawrence's earliest collaborators was Robert Alexander McCance (1898–1993), who had done three years' research at Cambridge with Sir Frederick Gowland Hopkins and came to King's College Hospital in 1926 to finish his medical studies. After qualifying in 1927, Mac, as he was known, helped Lawrence in the clinic for £30 a year. At that time, the carbohydrate value of foods was determined from American tables published in 1906 and based on raw foods. McCance showed that these were wrong because they did not distinguish available carbohydrate (starch and soluble sugars) from non-absorbable carbohydrates. The work was published in 1929 by McCance and Lawrence as a Medical Research Council special report, *The Carbohydrate Content of Foods*,[7,8] resulting in a major revision of the line ration diets, and indeed of all dietary schemes for diabetes. McCance is probably best known for his subsequent work in collaboration with Elsie Widdowson, whom he met in the hospital kitchen. Their *Chemical Composition of Foods* (1940) became the standard nutrition bible.[9]

Lawrence's work on the carbohydrate content of foods led to a delightful appeal letter in the *BMJ* in 1928 for bilberries and mulberries, which could not be obtained in the London shops.[10] 'Of course', he wrote, 'a gift of small amounts (say ½ lb) from a few sources would be still more gratefully received.' Later, searching for an artificial sweetener, Lawrence tested a commercial preparation of sorbitol (a polyhydric alcohol closely related to hexoses). Sorbitol was first used as a sweetener in 1929 and was thought to be particularly suitable for diabetics since it was not metabolized. Lawrence showed that it did not raise the blood sugar although it did cause 'intestinal irritation' (diarrhoea). He regarded it as an 'expensive luxury' and suggested that ordinary sugar with a little extra insulin was cheaper.[11] During the War, in 1940, the analysis of the protein content of earthworms, which might have been of dietetic value, was another example of Lawrence's ingenuity at this time of crisis.[12]

Actions of insulin

Lawrence's scientific curiosity led him to early and extensive studies of the mode of action of insulin both in animal and in human experiments. Already in 1924,[13] he had established that there was a difference between arterial and venous blood glucose levels, which influenced his experiments on a young diabetic man, which were reported in 1926.[14] He showed that the chief action of insulin was to lower blood glucose predominantly by converting it to glycogen, although he did not discount that it might also result in 'burning up' of glucose in the tissues. It also promoted conversion of glucose to fat. He attributed the insulin-enhancing effect of exercise[15] to depletion of glycogen stores, causing a 'glycogen vacuum'.

Incidentally, these observations led Lawrence, ever mindful of his patients, to offer very practical advice on management, not least that the dose of insulin should be reduced both before and after exercise or when patients left hospital[15] – advice often not heeded today. Even in those early days of insulin use, Lawrence observed that 'in winter more insulin sometimes seems necessary than in the summer, a result due either to increased calorific requirements in the cold or to more sedentary habits'.

Endocrine antagonism to insulin action

From the early 1900s, there was much interest in the interrelation of the endocrine glands, and this increased after the discovery of insulin. Hormones antagonistic to insulin, particularly from the pituitary but also from the adrenal and thyroid glands, were of special interest.[16] Lawrence found that an injection of pituitrin (a posterior pituitary extract marketed by Parke Davis) reduced the effectiveness of injected insulin,[17] and years later (in 1937) his friend and squash opponent Frank Young (1908–88) showed that injections of anterior pituitary extract into cats and dogs caused diabetes. On the basis of an antagonism between insulin and thyroid hormones, Lawrence used insulin unsuccessfully to treat exophthalmic goitre.[18] He also surmised (wrongly) that pituitary hormones might be responsible for retinopathy, and for the 'giant babies' occurring in diabetic pregnancies.[19] In later years, he noted that he had seen diabetes developing in many endocrine disorders, including acromegaly, Cushing's syndrome, and phaeochromocytoma, noting as well an association with Fröhlich's syndrome and Addison's disease.[20]

Insulin resistance

Studies of cases with severe insulin resistance were obviously relevant to Lawrence's attempts to understand the actions of insulin. As early as 1927, when he observed the effects of injecting diphtheria toxin into rabbits, he had speculated that excessive secretions from their adrenal and thyroid glands might be responsible[21] for the resulting insulin resistance. He could discover no explanation why one of his patients needed 220 units daily (and went into diabetic coma (ketoacidosis) when these were omitted)[22], or why another[23] needed 960 units before dying with heart failure. He thought there might be a failure of glycogen storage, perhaps due to lack of a coenzyme. He was well aware that infection could cause insulin resistance, and in his 1955 Lilly Lecture in the United States he recalled the 'dictum of a wise Indian doctor in the pre-insulin days who said that his fat and prosperous patients lived well enough with their diabetes for years until a vast carbuncle killed them in diabetic coma'.[24]

Lawrence's many clinical investigations were always conducted with meticulous measurements and recordings. They were at times bold and not always without hazard. On one occasion, he observed that after a pituitrin injection, some patients may go 'a ghastly grey colour ... fortunately their appearance was more terrifying than their feelings'.[17] In another instance, pituitrin injection four days after labour caused an epileptic convulsion. Lawrence seemed surprised that this patient 'objected to much investigation'.[19] On another occasion, he tried to find out how much insulin a 'brave volunteer' could take. This non-diabetic medical student was given increasing doses before breakfast on successive days. A dose of 40 units was tolerated without any symptoms.[17]

False remedies and abuses of insulin

Throughout his career, Lawrence responded very rapidly to supposedly new discoveries or false remedies, and always tested them himself.

The quest for an oral agent to replace insulin injections in the treatment of diabetes has never diminished. In 1925, a Dr Thomas Hollins of Chesterfield published a paper in the *BMJ* in which he claimed that 'raw gland seems to do all that insulin does in a diabetic case, while it is free from the grave risks attendant on the use of insulin'.[25] Lawrence demonstrated on himself that this was useless,[26] commenting that 'this was the worst experiment I ever tried on myself; to chew, swallow and keep down raw pancreas was a terrible and nauseating hardship, and after swallowing it felt as if the gullet was being digested. A serious return of sugar and acetone occurred with disproof of this nonsense.' George Graham and G. A. Harrison also found it to be useless with their patients. Another popular 'pancreatic preparation'[27] was widely advertised and used in the treatment of diabetes, although its effects represented no more than those of the accompanying diet. Lawrence brought the 'calamitous results' of using this agent to the readers of the *BMJ* in 1928,[27] especially after a patient developed ketoacidosis when his 'specialist' transferred treatment from insulin to this 'pancreatic preparation'. He beseeched that 'the public should be protected from this harm'.

A guanidine derivative Synthalin was produced in Germany in the 1920s and in 1926 the premier German diabetes specialist Oskar Minkowski wrote 'it is a momentous fact that the practical results exceeded all hopes ... now an insulin-like substance has actually been obtained that could help the great army of mild and medium severe diabetics.' Samples were sent to the MRC in early 1927 and their opinion was distinctly unfavourable.[28] Lawrence and others pointed out its toxicity in a discussion at the Royal Society of Medicine in 1928 and it was withdrawn in Britain in the same year.

In May 1927, a famous German diabetes specialist, Carl von Noorden, published an account of an oral pancreatic preparation, Glukhorment, that was said to have been obtained by 'strong tryptic digestion of fresh pancreas substance' and more crucially claimed not to contain Synthalin or related guanidine compounds.[29] It attracted a lot of attention – the 1928 Index Medicus contains 17 references to it compared with 44 for Synthalin. The Horment Company sent samples to Henry Dale at the National Institute for Medical Research in London and, when he and his colleague Harold Dudley analysed it, they found that it contained 1% of something that was chemically indistinguishable from synthalin.[30] At the request of the MRC Lawrence tested it on a 57-year-old man and a 12-year-old girl and found that it did lower the blood sugar but unsurprisingly had Synthalin-like side effects.[31]

Other agents included insulin phototungstate,[32] a liver extract,[33] and anterior pituitary extract,[34] all of which proved useless for those dependent on insulin injections. In 1937, the use of oral succinic acid was reported from Germany and elsewhere in Europe,[35] with the idea that it could replace insulin. Lawrence's scepticism was rapidly confirmed. An English newspaper had reported the use of succinic acid before its scientific publication, and some patients had pestered Lawrence to give them this new agent instead of insulin. Media exaggerations of spectacular novel 'treatments' are certainly not a new phenomenon.

Lawrence also campaigned against the misuse of insulin. In his 1936 lecture to the Medical Society of London,[36] he reported that it had been used for fattening the thin and combating anorexia, for improving cardiac efficiency, for treatment of peptic ulcers and skin ulcers, in the management of asthma and cancer and in the management of morphine addiction – the latter by Manfred Sakel, the inventor of insulin coma therapy for schizophrenia.

Types of diabetes

In 1951, Lawrence described several known causes of diabetes (pancreatectomy, hormonal, the diabète piqûre of Claude Bernard and alloxan-induced).[37] However, in most patients, the cause was unknown. Lawrence drew the distinction between those who suffered weight loss and ketosis as opposed to those who were ketosis-resistant and remained overweight ('lipoplethoric diabetes').

For many years, it had been suspected that there was more than one type of diabetes, but now the clinical scientific work of Lawrence established this distinction by one of his most important experiments with Joseph Bornstein. The background and methodology of Bornstein's method of measuring insulin was described in chapter 7.

Bornstein and Lawrence studied two groups of diabetic patients — 10 prone to ketosis and 37 non-ketosis prone: two publications followed showing beyond doubt the absence of circulating insulin in the former who we would now call type 1 diabetics and its presence in the 37 with what we would now call type 2 diabetes.[38,39]

In his 1955 Lilly Lecture in the USA, Lawrence consolidated this classification by defining the two principal types of diabetes as Type 1(lipoplethoric) and Type 2 (insulin dependent).[40] This crucial distinction of the two disorders with their distinctive features has undergone several descriptive revisions, but to this day determines fundamentally different approaches to treatment. Lawrence added Type 3 diabetes to his list, namely that of lipoatrophic diabetes, described in detail in chapter 7.

Lawrence suspected that insulin secretion in healthy nondiabetic individuals occurred not only in response to meals, but continued between them. He suggested a glucose-glycogen equilibrium as 'inherent as a heartbeat' indicating an element of liver regulation of blood glucose.[41] The quest for a single daily injection of long-acting insulin for the convenience of patients was first solved by Hagedorn in Denmark. Until 1936, insulin was simply known as 'insulin'. Now, with the introduction of variants, it acquired a range of names –'old', 'regular', 'ordinary', 'quick-acting' and 'soluble',[42] the last of these being a name that has continued in the UK to the present day. The development of long-acting insulins is described in detail in Chapter 7.

Diabetic coma (ketoacidosis)

Death was the expected outcome from diabetic coma (ketoacidosis) until 1922. However, when Joslin and colleagues reviewed their first 33 cases treated with insulin between January 1 1923 and April 1 1925 they reported that 31 had survived[43]. In a severe case the eyeballs were 'as soft as a jellyfish' and it was obvious that fluid was necessary. Nevertheless, according to Joslin et al, it needed to be given as gently and carefully 'as if the patient has just had a laparotomy'. The intravenous route had been used in the pre-insulin cases but in only one of the 33 post-insulin ones. Joslin wrote that, 'It is too risky. Too sudden a burden is thrown on a weak heart, and, furthermore, it is difficult to carry out because of the low blood pressure and small veins'. Fluid was sometimes given rectally but more often subcutaneously, subpectorally or into the thighs. Few hospitals in the USA or England achieved such good results as Joslin and in 1930 Lawrence recorded that the mortality was still high.[44] His description of a successful outcome in two of three 'desperate' cases marked a turning point, and he noted that even one year previously he was sure that they would all have died. His clinical description of these patients had identified dehydration and circulatory collapse as the prelude to death.[45] Lawrence's success was attributable to the use of large quantities of intravenous saline, complemented by gum acacia solution (which 'remains' in the vessels) together with large doses of insulin: 'One or two pints is not enough, and frequently three to six pints must be given over one to two hours to restore the circulation'. Additional circulatory support was considered essential, using adrenaline with strophanthin [46]. Caffeine was always given subcutaneously in 5-grain doses every hour for the first few hours, often supplemented by a coffee enema. In one patient he gave 9 pints of hypertonic saline (seven intravenously) in 18 hours and noted that even after so much she only passed a few ounces of urine. He seems to have been emboldened to give so much fluid by tropical medicine experts who recommended a pint every five minutes intravenously in patients with cholera. In 1936 he repeated his view that large amounts of intravenous saline were necessary in patients with profound dehydration.[47]

The dose of insulin to be given was disputed. In 1948, Robert H. Micks (1895–1972), Professor of Pharmacology at the Royal College of Surgeons in Ireland, published a paper in the *BMJ* in which he recommended an initial 100 units for patients in precoma, 500 units for true coma and then 100 units intravenously every 15 minutes (*sic*) until there were clinical signs of improvement.[48] The article was heavily criticized in the correspondence columns. Lawrence and Oakley pointed out that Micks had not produced any evidence (his paper was a review, which drew heavily on the work of Joslin's associate Howard Root) and questioned his assertion that improvement would be seen in 15 minutes after a subcutaneous injection.[49] They presented three recent cases of their own in which the *total* doses needed to restore the patients to full consciousness were 124, 142 and 196 units, and suggested that larger doses would have caused hypoglycaemia. They did admit to sometimes giving large doses, but only as a desperate measure in cases of circulatory collapse, in which they thought that most of the insulin was wasted anyway.

In later years,[47] Lawrence's opinion was that diabetic coma should 'theoretically never occur', and should no longer be a cause of death – yet it still sometimes occurred, and he reported a case where insulin 'had been criminally stopped for two days on account of vomiting'.[50] It is interesting that, even by 1952, Lawrence was doubtful about the existence of diabetic coma without ketosis.[51] Underlying all his scientific observations, however, he was always making helpful clinical observations: if a coma patient was incontinent, why not test for ketosis by sprinkling ferric chloride powder on the wet sheets![52]

In 1931, Lawrence wrote a case report in the *BMJ* of 'the diabetic acute abdomen' which had been described in the American literature but not in a British journal. The 31-year-old patient had severe abdominal pain and rigidity, together with a white cell count of 51,000. There did not seem to be any way of distinguishing between appendicitis or a perforated gastric ulcer and the diabetic acute abdomen. Lawrence wrote that, 'had we not known that a high leucocytosis may be present [in diabetic coma] without any septic focus, the high count would have demanded immediate operation.' In an article on rare clinical manifestations in diabetic coma and precoma, he admitting to having misdiagnosed two cases of fulminating appendicitis as the diabetic acute abdomen. In the same article, he described a unique case in which the patient was so violent as to need physical restraint and had to be given chloroform to achieve intravenous access.[51]

Hypoglycaemia

The problems of abnormally low blood glucose levels (hypoglycaemia or 'hypo') emerged as soon as insulin was introduced, and Lawrence's early descriptions lean heavily on his own experiences. Both *The Diabetic Life*[53] and *The Diabetic ABC*[54] contain excellent descriptions of the clinical features and correct management. Indeed, Lawrence himself experienced his own first episode of hypoglycaemia just 6 hours after his first insulin injection. He attributed the early warning symptoms of hypoglycaemia to stimulation of the autonomic nervous system, noting that they preceded the development of neurological features. Writing years later,[55] he presented the new observation that after between 5 and 10 years of diabetes, or when using the new long-acting insulin, protamine zinc insulin, early warning symptoms may diminish or even disappear, resulting in the early development of neurological features, including diminished cognition and double vision, with potentially devastating consequences.[56] Lawrence could not explain this change, but indicated ways in which patients might avoid hypoglycaemia in the first place.

Pregnancy

Lawrence had a longstanding interest in diabetic pregnancy and by 1948 said that he had followed 200 cases before 1941,[57] and 141 between 1941 and 1948. It is often said that insulin revolutionized the outlook in diabetic pregnancy. In fact, in the first decade after insulin, pregnancy in diabetic women was uncommon and the benefit of insulin was almost exclusively on maternal mortality. At a meeting at the Royal Society of Medicine in 1927, Arnold (later Sir Arnold) Walker (1897–1968), at the time an obstetric registrar, reported that he had only found one case in the records of the Middlesex Hospital in the previous 23 years.[58] Since the discovery of insulin, he could only find 18 in the literature, with a maternal mortality rate of 10% and a fetal mortality rate of 27%. He concluded that 'The administration of insulin has entirely altered the outlook for the better in cases of pregnancy complicated with diabetes, as indeed it has done in diabetes generally.' In the discussion, Lawrence said that during the previous 3 years he had investigated 24 pregnant women in whom persistent glycosuria had been discovered on routine examination. In 16, it was due to a low renal threshold for glucose and these patients did well without any change of diet. His results in patients with true diabetes were not very good, and he suggested that the pregnancy should be terminated if 'a very heavy ketosis or hydramnios occurred, or if the foetus showed signs of being unduly large'.[60]

At the next meeting of the Royal Society of Medicine,[59] Lawrence described a woman who had had 11 pregnancies: 5 live births before developing diabetes, followed by 6 further pregnancies with only one survivor (weighing 12 lb 6 oz), followed by disappearance of her diabetes. He was clearly baffled by a form of diabetes so 'unlike pancreatic diabetes'. Based on other evidence that the woman had a pituitary tumour, he considered that pituitrin might be at fault, and indeed later questioned whether it might be the cause of the 'giant babies' associated with diabetic pregnancy.[60] Another early publication[61] described a diabetic patient with a twin pregnancy where insulin requirements rose initially but after 28 weeks fell considerably, only to rise again after delivery: his ingenious suggestion that fetal insulin might be contributing to control of maternal diabetes could not be upheld.

After enticing Wilfred Oakley from Bart's in 1938, Lawrence seems to have transferred the care of pregnant diabetics to his colleague. In 1942, they presented a lengthy and definitive treatise on the outcome and management of diabetic pregnancy – a paper that served as a prelude to many years of research at King's leading eventually to vast improvements. They noted that maternal mortality had virtually disappeared, yet fetal loss remained 'remarkably high' – 33% in their series of 54 pregnancies, but ranging from just 23% in those with optimal care to 70% in those without any. They concluded that 'if a pregnant diabetic is allowed to go to term without special supervision either the baby tends to be over-sized and is often stillborn or, should a live child be delivered, death within 24 to 48 hours of delivery is not uncommon, no obvious cause being present'.[60] As a result, their key recommendation was that delivery should be by induction or caesarean section at 36–38 weeks – a practice that continued for many years thereafter.

Overall results at King's remained poor until 1958, when Oakley and Peel[62] decided to admit all pregnant diabetics at 32 weeks and deliver them at 36 weeks. The original reason for admission, during which the woman was in bed for 20 hours a day, was to improve blood flow though the uterus. However, it also meant that the diabetes could be better controlled and monitored. Results improved substantially with this new regimen, with a fall in fetal mortality rate from 25% to 13%.

Lawrence's teaching on marriage and pregnancy in diabetics changed considerably in his lifetime. In the 1920s, his advice was dominated by consideration of pregnancy and the inheritance of diabetes. In the earlier editions of *The Diabetic Life*,[53] he wrote that 'marriage is not dangerous to men ... women must be cautioned of the danger to themselves as well as to their offspring. ... The balance of opinion is that, while marriage cannot justly be forbidden, pregnancy is highly inadvisable in all but the exceptional case.' Until the mid 1930s, 'Pregnancy is usually inadvisable' remained the advice. By 1937, a much more positive approach was taken, with Lawrence writing, 'Many cases have been successfully conducted through pregnancy by the use of insulin and usually a normal child is born.'

Case histories

Lawrence was President of the Endocrine Section of the Royal Society of Medicine in 1950, and regularly attended its meetings. His vast clinical experience enabled him to describe and publish reports on unusual case histories, often accompanied by perceptive vignettes of his patients. Of one patient, he wrote that 'she was a spirited and clever young woman who led the wildest of diabetic lives, travelling all over the world on insulin varying from 20 to 80 units per day, often loaded with sugar and ketones, precomatose from short supplies of insulin in the tropics, and a perfect candidate for retinal and other complications'.[57] Ultimately, Lawrence's main goal was always for the benefit of his patients, especially the 'individual patient',[63] while observing that most of the difficulties in management occurred in those whom he described as either 'careless' or 'unintelligent' compared with those who were 'cooperative'. Some examples of his keen sense of clinical observation, often presenting new insights into the nature of diabetes itself, are described below in chronological order:

1930. Lawrence described a regimen of glucose and insulin that enabled surgery to be undertaken, bearing in mind that, before insulin, the presence of diabetes was regarded as a bar to any operation. He noted a mortality rate of 13% of 163 operations – alarming now, but remarkably low in the preantibiotic days of 1930.[64]

1931. Lawrence and McCance described an 18-day-old baby who developed transient diabetes needing insulin treatment. The baby developed four inexplicable areas of necrosis or gangrene, all of which healed, and a normal, non-diabetic child eventually left the hospital. The paper contained an extensive review of the literature on diabetes under age 1 year and concluded that only 26 definite cases had been reported since 1850.[65]

1933. A case of diabetes mellitus and diabetes insipidus both occurring in one patient was reported by Lawrence and McCance, with the conclusion that this was an entirely fortuitous combination of disorders. Insulin and pituitrin (posterior pituitary extract) were mixed together in the same syringe, with the comment that 'it is fortunate that two such serious diseases can be controlled as easily as one in the same patient – although perhaps not so cheaply!'.[66]

1935. Lawrence reported a family with a history of diabetes associated with haemochromatosis, a rare condition 'probably due to an inborn error of iron metabolism'.[67] The striking male predominance of this condition led him to suggest (erroneously) that 'like haemophilia' it was a sex-linked hereditary disease. His subsequent report on 12 cases showed that treatment with insulin resulted in normal activity for several years, noting at the same time their tendency to insulin resistance.[68] More details are presented in Chapter 7.

1936. The abnormality of the glucose tolerance test known as the lag storage curve had been described and named by Hugh Maclean, Professor of Medicine at St Thomas's. In a 1936 paper, Lawrence noted how often it occurred after gastroenterostomy and concluded that it was due to rapid intestinal absorption of glucose and did not indicate any abnormality of carbohydrate metabolism.[69] He pointed out that the nomenclature was misleading, since the curve was not slow or lagging but rather sharp and steeple-like. He suggested the name 'oxyhyperglycaemia', which, in his words, 'has the double merit of good description and good Greek'.

1941. Lawrence and Kate Madders argued that since pituitary activity increased in women at the menopause while oestrogen levels declined, treatment with oestrogen preparations might ameliorate the diabetes. Starting in 1939, they had intended to treat 50 women, but had only managed to study 5 before war intervened. The women were treated with 4 mg stilboestrol a day for 8 weeks without any discernible effect on their glucose control.[70]

1942. Lawrence described his 'mixed feelings' on treating three 'mongol idiots' (Down's syndrome) with insulin.[71] He clearly did so reluctantly, writing that 'however much one might consider such therapy wasted and displaced this has not been the parental attitude'. He reported graciously that all three children responded well and their management had not been unduly difficult over between 2 and 10 years. The huge societal change of attitude to disability since that time places this case report in a darker era of history.

1947. In a Population Survey, 778 male army recruits were found to have glycosuria on routine testing and were referred to Lawrence. Glucose tolerance tests established that while 65% had renal glycosuria, as many as 18% had diabetes.[72]

1949. The presence of haemorrhages in the eyes of patients with diabetes had been known for many years. Lawrence reassuringly pointed out that some patients never developed retinopathy. Furthermore, he observed that lesions may appear and disappear[73] – an observation that 'ophthalmologists are apt to disbelieve because they do not watch patients for years and years'.[73] His colleague Theodore Whittington, examining Lawrence himself in 1951, reported that he had no retinal haemorrhages even after 31 years of diabetes.[74] Further observations on retinopathy are in Chapter 7.

1954. Responding to an article in the *BMJ* on pancreatic cancer, Lawrence wrote to point out that the surgeon authors had failed to mention that diabetes could be the first symptom.[75] He admitted that it was rare, but said he had seen it in 12 cases where diabetes began between 3 and 18 months before the appearance of jaundice. He suggested that when an elderly diabetic continued to lose weight in spite of adequate treatment, one should suspect cancer of the pancreas.

1956. Some 34 years after the introduction of insulin, Lawrence participated in an early trial to test the hypoglycaemic action of an oral sulphonylurea derivative, namely BZ55, otherwise known as carbutamide.[76] The report from King's was published jointly with his successor Dr Wilfred Oakley, and clearly demonstrated the effectiveness of BZ55 in those over 40 years of age without ketonuria (type 2 diabetes) and its ineffectiveness in younger ketotic patients (type 1 diabetes),[77] in accordance with results obtained in other trials. Although this particular agent proved too toxic for clinical use, it nevertheless opened a new era of diabetes treatment that must have thrilled Lawrence after witnessing so many failures.

Lawrence made numerous other clinical observations on diverse topics, including diabetes and multiple pregnancies; haematuria; low renal threshold for glucose; eosinophilia and insulin therapy; postoperative acidosis; effect of infection on insulin action; and acromegaly. He published many insightful case reports, describing, often for the first time, the great majority of problems that might arise over a lifetime of diabetes.

Education

The training of the diabetic in his life-long creed is the most important part of his treatment. It is also the part that is most likely to be neglected through lack of time and opportunity.

The more a diabetic knows and understands his disease, the better he is able to enjoy good health and lead a normal life in spite of it – in other words, to conquer it.

It should be the object of all treatment to enable a diabetic to lead a normal and varied life, and to forget all about his disease except at meal times.

Lawrence's principal books were *The Diabetic Life*,[53] which ran to 17 editions from 1925 to 1965, and *The Diabetic ABC: A Practical Book for Patients and Nurses*,[54] a shorter, practical guide, which also ran to a large number of editions from the 1st in 1929 to the 14th in 1967. A small concise booklet entitled *Almost All About Diabetes*[77] in the 'Family Doctor' series, published by the British Medical Association, was a summary of all aspects of clinical diabetes, culminating in a list of 32 questions on what every diabetic should know. For example:

Do you ever boil your syringe to keep it sterile?

and

How long does an insulin needle last before it must be changed?

the answers being, respectively:

Not necessary; syringe may break and needle blunted

and

With proper care and skilful injections, three months or even longer

The 1st and 17th editions of *The Diabetic Life* have a lot in common, showing the care with which it was first written. A review of the 14th edition sums up the important role this book played in the care of diabetes:

This hardy and well-tried perennial ... has served as guide, philosopher and friend to a whole generation of diabetics. Books may come and go, but Lawrence's 'Diabetic Life' apparently goes on for ever. This is because it is an essentially clear and practical book, founded on its author's unrivalled experience of diabetes and diabetics.

With this book, it was possible for the general practitioner, the hospital resident and the intelligent patient to undertake the general management of diabetes. It is not known how many drafts Lawrence needed, but, according to his son Adam, he spent most evenings writing at his desk. A lot of time must also have been spent in proof reading – for example, in the first edition of *The Diabetic Life* in 1925, which contains 161 pages packed with information, there are only two errata. The book was translated into French, Spanish, Dutch, Italian and Swedish.

Lawrence was interested in medical education and regretted the lack of training of the teachers of medicine and how teaching hospital appointments failed to consider this important.[78] His philosophy was that 'though bad teachers cannot be made good ones, moderate ability can be improved, and even the born teacher, too'. He listed some sins of lecturing, including inaudible whispering and mumbling, humming and hawing, distracting mannerisms, and complicated diagrams with no explanation:

Surely we could all be helped and improved in these varied venial sins by the elocutionists, the educationists, and the friendly criticism of our peers, especially at an early and malleable stage.

He also felt that it was essential in both the practice of medicine and teaching to develop a systematized method of thought:

Some logic, philosophy, psychology of teaching process would help to develop and sharpen the mental acuteness and awareness.

How many times has it been said:

The medical curriculum must be changed and be pruned of its impossible burden on pure memory, but it is equally important that the student should acquire a definite basic mental process of thought as a stand-by for ever.

He deplored the tendency to divide medical education into the theoretical or intellectually educative, to be mainly the concern of academic whole-time intellectual highbrows and research workers, and the vocational or technical, the concern mainly of part-time clinical practitioners of clinical medicine:

Nothing, I think, could be more unreal or disastrous. Both aspects must be welded into a sound fundamental training from which all later activities must constantly stem.

For general practitioners, Lawrence deplored training courses containing too many subjects in a short time, and advocated a specialized, intensive approach on one subject over a longer period of time.[79]

In his book *Clinical Medicine: Some Principles of Thinking, Learning and Teaching*, published in 1954,[80] he despaired about the use of the English language and thought that spelling was often extremely bad:

This, I suppose, is not by itself a clear sign of a poor brain capacity, but merely a lack of careful education. Poor writing, bad grammatical construction, negligible or wrong punctuation, the lack of clear sentences and the absence or over-use of paragraphs is an indication of a disorderly illogical mind. And an illegible handwriting is, and deserves to be, a severe handicap, not only in examinations but right throughout life whenever written communication is necessary. Many doctors' letters I give up in despair, as life is too short to spend half an hour in deciphering them.

Conclusions

Lawrence began researching the nature of diabetes and its treatment even before he himself started insulin. He never stopped searching until his death nearly half a century later. He wanted to discover the best mode of care for every individual patient, and his primary goal was always to 'relieve suffering'.[73] Whenever innovation was in the air, he set out to confirm or refute its validity, at the same time hounding the press and others for preposterous exaggeration. In innumerable case descriptions and letters to journals, he made a host of original clinical observations – and more recent texts have little to add. Throughout his life, he was always conscious of the situation before insulin, and in one of his last publications, in 1963,[81] he reviewed the outcome of 90 of his patients over 20–40 years, commenting that 'it was a joy to see how quickly such patients, myself included, were rebuilt'. He could not resist writing one last communication in 1967,[82] just one year before he died and after developing a left hemiplegia, describing the sensation of 'neuritis' that had developed on his left side with similar features to the 'neuritis' that troubled him before starting insulin in 1923.

Among Lawrence's many original medical and scientific contributions, the carbohydrate content of foods, the differentiation of what we now call type 1 and type 2 diabetes, the recognition of extreme insulin resistance, and the principle of educating all patients with diabetes to become self-sufficient will remain lasting legacies.

Of the many tributes paid to Lawrence, the value of his researches was never better expressed than in a letter of 1931 from Sir Walter Fletcher (1873–1933) at the Medical Research Council when he wrote:[83]

You helped greatly in our early work upon insulin, and yet, if insulin had become available a few months later, you would have been dead for want of it. Your work, and its success, has been due to a curious and very happy stroke of fate. I say this, though I admit the poverty of the expression 'fate'.

References

1. National Archive. Correspondence between GA Harrison and the Medical Research Council (1922–1923): 1.
2. Harrison GA, Lawrence RD. Diastase in blood and urine in diabetes mellitus. *Br Med J* 1923; **i**: 317–19.
3. Lawrence RD. Types of human diabetes. *Br Med J* 1951; **i**: 373–5.
4. Lawrence RD. A diabetic diet: the line ration scheme. *Br Med J* 1925; **i**: 261.
5. *Food Tables*. Privately printed, 1924.
6. Harrison GA, Lawrence RD. *Food Tables: Compiled Particularly for the Use in Treatment of Diabetes Mellitus*, 2nd edn. London: HH Skinner, 1924.
7. Lawrence RD, McCance RA. *The Carbohydrate Content of Foods*. London: HMSO, 1929.
8. Lawrence RD, McCance RA. New analyses of carbohydrate foods and their application to diabetic diets. *Br Med J* 1929; **ii**: 241.
9. McCance RA, Widdowson E. *The Chemical Composition of Foods*. Medical Research Council: Special Report Series No. 235, 1940.
10. Lawrence RD. A request for bilberries and mulberries. *Br Med J* 1928; **ii**: 474.
11. Payne WW, Lawrence RD, McCance RA. Sorbitol (Sionon) for diabetics. *Lancet* 1933; **ii**: 1257–8.
12. Lawrence RD, Millar HR. Protein content of earthworms. *Nature* 1945; **155**: 517.
13. Lawrence RD. Effect of insulin on the sugar content of arterial and venous blood in diabetes. *Br Med J* 1924; **i**: 516–17.
14. Lawrence RD. The action of insulin in glycogen formation and its therapeutic application. *Q J Med* 1926; **20**: 69–86.
15. Lawrence RD. The effect of exercise on insulin action in diabetes. *Br Med J* 1926; **i**: 648–50.
16. Lawrence RD, McCance RA. The effect of starvation, phloridzin, thyroid, adrenaline, insulin and pituitrin on the distribution of glycogen in the rat. *Biochem J* 1931; **25**: 570–8.
17. Hewlett RFL, Lawrence RD. The effect of pituitrin and insulin on blood sugar, their antagonism and the mode of its action. *Br Med J* 1925; **i**: 998–1002.
18. Lawrence, RD. Four cases of exophthalmic goitre treated with insulin. Brit Med J 1924;2: 753–755.
19. Lawrence, RD. Association of multiple pregnancies with diabetes of suggested pituitary origin. *Proc Roy Soc Med* 1927; **21**: 9–16.

20. Lawrence RD. Cases. Diabetes mellitus with obesity and acromegaly. Haemochromatosis. *Proc Roy Soc Med* 1950; **43**: 355–358.
21. Lawrence RD, Buckley OB. The inhibition of insulin action by toxaemias and its explanation. The effect of diphtheria toxin on blood-sugar and insulin action in rabbits. *Brit J Exp Path* 1927; **8**: 58–75.
22. Lawrence RD. Studies of an insulin-resistant diabetic. *Quart J Med* 1928; **21**: 359–369.
23. Lawrence RD, Clay RD. An insulin-resistant diabetic. *Brit Med J* 1935; **1**: 697–698.
24. Lawrence RD. Three types of human diabetes. *Ann Int Med* 1955; **43**: 1199–1208.
25. Hollins TJ. Treatment of diabetes by raw fresh gland (pancreas). *Brit Med J* 1925;1:503–504.
26. Lawrence RD. Raw pancreas by mouth compared with insulin. *Brit Med J* 1925; **1**: 1108.
27. Lawrence RD. Oral administration of pancreatic preparations. *Brit Med J* 1928; **1**: 875.
28. Graham G, Poulton EP. The synthalin treatment of diabetes: preliminary report to the Medical Research Council. *Lancet* 1927;2:517–521.
29. Von Noorden C. Glukhorment, a new antiglycosuric substance formed in the body. *Klin Wchnschr* 1927; 22: 1041–1043.
30. Dale HH, Dudley HW. The active constituent of the preparation called 'glukhorment'. *Br Med J* 1927; **2**: 1027–1029.
31. Diabetes Mellitus Treated with Glukhorment. *Br Med J* 1927;ii: 1184–5
32. Lawrence RD. Insulin phosphotungstate by mouth. *Lancet* 1931; **1**: 184–185.
33. Lawrence RD. The action of liver preparations on diabetes. *Lancet* 1930; **ii**: 1179–80.
34. Lawrence RD, Young FG. Oral anterior pituitary extract (Collip) in diabetes. *Lancet* 1940; **ii**: 709–710.
35. Lawrence RD, McCance RA, Archer, N. Succinic acid treatment of diabetic ketosis. *Br Med J* 1937; **ii**: 214.
36. Graham G, Lawrence RD. The use and abuse of insulin. *Trans Med Soc Lond* 1936; **59**: 52–65.
37. Lawrence RD. Types of human diabetes. *Br Med J* 1951; **i**: 373–5.
38. Bornstein J, Lawrence RD.Two types of diabetes, with and without available plasma insulin. *Brit Med J* 1951; **1**: 732.
39. Bornstein J, Lawrence RD. Plasma insulin in human diabetes mellitus. *Brit Med J* 1951; **2**: 1541–1544.
40. Lawrence RD. Three types of human diabetes. *Ann Intern Med* 1955; **43**: 1199–208.
41. Lawrence RD, Archer N. Some experiments with protamine insulinate. *Br Med J* 1936; **i**: 747–8.
42. Lawrence RD, Archer N. Zinc protamine insulin; a clinical trial of the new preparation. *Br Med J* 1937; **i**: 487–491.
43. Joslin EP, Root HF, White P. Diabetic coma and its treatment. *Med Clin N Amer* 1925; **8**: 1873–1919.
44. Lawrence RD. The treatment of desperate cases of diabetic coma. *Brit Med J* 1930; **i**: 690–692.
45. Lawrence RD. Insulin therapy in diabetes mellitus. *Brit Med J* 1927; **2**: 1021–1022.
46. Lawrence RD. Treatment of diabetic coma. *Brit Med J* 1929; **1**: 107–109.
47. Lawrence RD. Treatment of diabetic coma. *Br Med J* 1936; **ii**: 81–2.
48. Micks RH. Diabetic coma. *Br Med J* 1948; **ii**: 200–3.
49. Lawrence RD, Oakley WG. Diabetic coma. *Br Med J* 1948; **ii**: 310.
50. Lawrence RD. Rare clinical manifestations in diabetic coma and precoma. *Diabetes* 1956; **5**: 484–6.
51. Lawrence RD, Oakley WG, Martin MM. Diabetic acidosis without ketonuria. *Lancet* 1952; **i**: 923.

52. Lawrence RD. Acetone tests on the bed-sheets in diabetic coma. *Br Med J* 1954; **i**: 336.
53. Lawrence RD. *The Diabetic Life*, 1st edn. London: J & A Churchill, 1925; 17th edn, 1965.
54. Lawrence RD. *The Diabetic ABC: A Practical Book for Patients and Nurses*, 1st edn, London: HK Lewis, 1929; 14th edn, 1967.
55. Lawrence RD. Insulin hypoglycaemia: changes in nervous manifestations. *Lancet* 1941; **ii**: 602.
56. Lawrence RD. Increase in hypoglycaemia. *Br Med J* 1942; **i**: 802–3.
57. Lawrence RD. Acute retinopathy without hyperpiesis in diabetic pregnancy. *Br J Ophthalmol* 1948; **32**: 461–5.
58. Walker A. Diabetes mellitus and pregnancy. *Proc R Soc Med* 1927–28; **21**: 377–85.
59. Lawrence RD. Association of multiple pregnancies with diabetes of suggested pituitary origin. *Proc R Soc Med* 1927; **21**: 243–50.
60. Lawrence RD, Oakley W. Pregnancy and diabetes. *Q J Med* 1942; **41**: 45–75.
61. Lawrence RD. Improvement of diabetes in pregnant woman due to foetal insulin. *Q J Med* 1929; **22**: 191–202.
62. Peel JH. Diabetes in pregnancy. *Proc R Soc Med* 1963; **56**: 1009–11.
63. Lawrence RD. Diabetes: with special reference to high carbohydrate diets. *Br Med J* 1933; **ii**: 517–21.
64. Lawrence RD. Surgery in diabetes. *Br Med J* 1930; **ii**: 1002–3.
65. Lawrence RD, McCance RA. Gangrene in an infant associated with temporary diabetes. *Arch Dis Child* 1931; **6**: 343–56.
66. Lawrence RD, McCance RA. Diabetes mellitus and insipidus associated in one case. *Lancet* 1933; **i**: 76–7.
67. Lawrence RD. Haemochromatosis and heredity. *Lancet* 1935; **ii**: 1055–6.
68. Lawrence RD. The prognosis of haemochromatosis. *Lancet* 1936; **ii**: 1171–2.
69. Lawrence RD. Glycosuria of 'lag storage' type: an explanation. *Br Med J* 1936; **i**: 526–7.
70. Lawrence RD, Madders K. Human diabetes treated with oestrogens. *Lancet* 1941; **i**: 601–2.
71. Lawrence RD. Three diabetic mongol idiots. *Br Med J* 1942; **i**: 695.
72. Keeping LA, Lawrence RD. Glycosuria in recruits: incidence and classification. *Lancet* 1947; **i**: 901–3.
73. Lawrence RD. Insulin therapy: successes and problems. *Lancet* 1949; **ii**: 401–5.
74. Lawrence RD. Discussion on diabetic retinopathy. *Proc R Soc Med* 1951; **44**: 742–3.
75. Lawrence RD. Diabetes as first sign of pancreatic carcinoma. *Br Med J* 1954; **ii**: 593.
76. Hunt JA, Oakley WG, Lawrence RD. Clinical trial of the new oral hypoglycaemic agent BZ55. *Br Med J* 1956; **ii**: 445–448.
77. Lawrence RD. *Almost All About Diabetes*. London: British Medical Association, 1949.
78. Lawrence RD. The training of clinical teachers. *Br Med J* 1950; **ii**: 481–4.
79. Lawrence RD. Adult education for the GP. *Br Med J* 1955; **ii**: 681.
80. Lawrence RD. *Clinical Medicine: Some Principles of Thinking, Learning and Teaching*. London: HK Lewis, 1954.
81. Lawrence RD. Treatment of 90 severe diabetics with soluble insulin for 20–40 years: effect of diabetic control on complications. *Br Med J* 1963; **ii**: 1634–5.
82. Lawrence RD. Hemiplegia in a diabetic producing unilateral peripheral neuritis and hypoglycaemic attacks. *Lancet* 1967; **i**: 1321–2.
83. National Archive. Correspondence between GA Harrison and the Medical Research Council (1922–1923): 7.

CHAPTER 13

The Later Years

Thank you for teaching us how to live in joy and happiness.

Inscription on a gift from the IDF to Lawrence

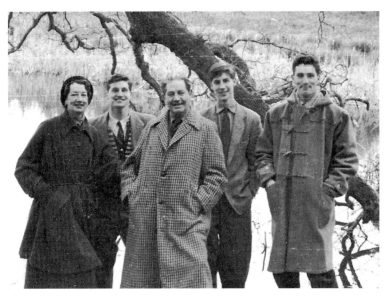

The Lawrence family at Frensham Ponds in 1953: Anna, Adam, Dan and Rob.
The photograph was taken by Rob's wife, Clover.

In 1956, Lawrence was awarded the Fothergillian Gold Medal of the Medical Society of London. It was first presented in 1787 and, apart from a short interval from 1803 to 1824, has continued until the present day. It is:

awarded to a British subject, either for the best essay on some branch of Practical Medicine or Practical Surgery proposed by the Trustees (MSL Council) or for a literary work on some branch of Practical Medicine or Practical Surgery published within a period of 5 years prior to the award of the prize.[1]

This was from a legacy instituted by Dr Anthony Fothergill, who left £500 to endow an annual or triennial medal on the subject of 'Insanity; Pulmonary Consumption; Cancer; Dropsy (particularly of the brain); or Croup'. Other circumstances were left to the Society's discretion, which is presumably why none of the distinguished individuals who have received the Fothergillian Award has had to produce an essay, or work on any of the subjects that Dr Fothergill specified.[2] Lawrence received his gold medal for *The Diabetic Life*, by then in its 15th edition with over 50,000 copies sold. He became the 62nd recipient of the medal, joining an illustrious gallery, including his friends and contemporaries Sir Henry Dale and Sir Harold Himsworth.

Lawrence, with his son Dan, travelled to Iceland in June 1957 to deliver a lecture at a medical conference and to spend some time sightseeing and fishing. They looked at waterfalls, glaciers, geysers and volcanoes while marvelling at the midnight sun, and enjoyed five days of fishing with their host, Dr Albertson. Lawrence reported to Anna that, beneath a waterfall:

I got a 4 lb salmon, then Dan a 9½ pounder. It rushed down the rapids so the excited Dr thinking Dan would lose it, grabbed his rod and between them it was landed. Later I got two more on a fly and had a long and really thrilling fight down 80 yards of rushing water – adrenaline as well as the fish running hard! Four salmon in a morning seems to be the record this year – Ha Ha the Lawrences! These small fish, lovely to eat, have been put in a deep freeze so we should bring something home. We slept a little this afternoon, then visited a Health Centre, dined out alone, and now early to bed.

Lawrence appreciated the care given by his son on their Icelandic jaunt:

Dan is looking after me v well. Valeting, washing, brushing my hair and smartening me – jolly good.

In October 1957, shortly before his retirement from Kings, Lawrence suffered a serious stroke, from which he made a remarkable recovery, although he was left with dense paralysis in the left arm and leg. He had been a heavy smoker throughout his life and many of the group photographs at medical congresses show all the doctors holding cigarettes, as was common at the time. After his stroke, he not only gave up smoking but insisted that no-one should smoke in his presence.

After a long convalescent break in Portugal with Anna, followed by several months at home, he resumed active practice, and was able to

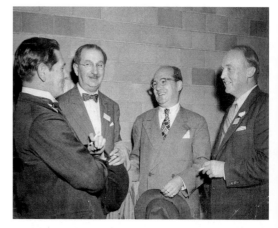

Lawrence (left) and Charles Best (right) at a medical conference, taking a smoking break.

travel to meetings, where he became renowned for sitting in the front row and asking penetrating questions or throwing in a contribution to illustrate a point from his own vast experience. He was, however, unable to attend the Third IDF Congress in Düsseldorf, where his presidency came to an end, and he was elected an Honorary President. In recognition of his strong leadership, a silver writing block was presented to him by Dr Frank on behalf of the IDF, inscribed 'Thank you for teaching us how to live in joy and happiness.'

Lawrence although in failing health, went to some subsequent congresses. He travelled to Toronto for the Fifth IDF Congress in July 1964, where he was honoured by the University with an Honorary Degree of Doctor of Law. Charles Best was unwell at the time, but, accompanied by Adam, Lawrence made the journey to the steamy hot city, and survived the journey well despite a heavy thunderstorm en route. At a special Convocation of the University, on a hot evening, he entered the hall crowded with many old friends from all over the world, escorted by Adam and walking with a stick. Everyone watched with bated breath as he awkwardly negotiated the several steps up to the platform, where he sat with Joseph J. Hoet, his old friend and colleague, and a fellow diabetic, Dr Randall Sprague (1906–90) of the Mayo Clinic in Rochester, Minnesota, who were to be similarly honoured. After the citation had been read, Jackson reported that Lawrence:

> rose to his feet, threw down his stick and walked (shuffled might be more accurate) to receive his certificate, and then back to his seat, while the audience loudly applauded. It was a typical gesture of frustration in his present circumstance, and of courage to overcome all that life could throw at him.

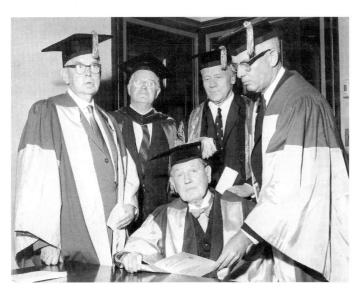

Toronto University, July 1964. The Chancellor, F. C. A. Jeanneret (left) and the Dean of the Faculty, V.W. Bladen (back left), with Lawrence, Joseph Hoet and Randall Sprague receiving their honorary degrees for diabetes research

During the 1950s, Lawrence found himself baffled by some of the scientific papers that were being presented at congresses. In an undated letter to Anna he wrote:

Today's two sessions were intense, highbrow and confusing to me. Some intensely chemical papers I could hardly understand and nobody seemed to have a rational explanation of what these difficult experiments mean. Had our chairs been less hard many of us would have slept soundly.

The following day he reported:

Countless obscure lectures with obscure meanings, not only for me but most. Last night's dinner with the Canadians, good in food but poor in wit.

In January 1955, he was moved to write to the *BMJ* on the topic of scientific terms:[3]

For those of us who spend a few week-end hours in trying to keep up to date in new medical discoveries about which we know nothing, it would be most helpful if a preliminary paragraph introduced us as simply as possible to the subject. For instance, I have to-day battled with articles on phenylketonuria[4] (Journal, January 8, p. 57) and byssinosis[5] (p. 65) without ever getting my ignorant feet on the ground for a good start in understanding them. I have always told myself and my juniors to kick off with a simple explanatory paragraph relating the past to the new when writing about specialized novelties. I hope you, Sir, will insist on this when your authors tend to neglect it.

Wilfred Oakley later summed of this aspect of his colleague:

Both in his teaching and writing Lawrence aimed at simplicity of thought and expression; he sometimes underrated the intelligence of his audience.

In 1958 Lawrence suggested that a 'Lawrence Research Prize Fund' worth £50 be established at KCH for work on diabetes or a closely related subject. This was duly set up and is open to any pre-clinical student awaiting entry to King's College Hospital, or any student or member of the staff of the Hospital, provided that 'he or she shall not have been qualified for more than seven years.' Lawrence was proud of the prize fund which has been awarded each year since 1959. Further prizes in recognition of his work came after his death. In 1973 the British Diabetic Association established the RD Lawrence lectureship, which is awarded to a researcher under the age of 45. An annually competitive scheme, the RD Lawrence Fellowship, was established by the BDA in 1976. It is a career development fellowship which enables postdoctoral researchers to establish their independence in diabetes research.

In September 1958, Lawrence and Anna moved to a large mansion flat overlooking a beautiful communal garden at Sheffield Terrace off Church Street in Kensington. It had become increasingly difficult for him to climb stairs, and they were delighted with the move. Anna noted on their change-of-address card that it was almost like living in the country and that Lawrence walked in the garden every morning before he went to work.

On 27 May 1959, a dinner was held in the Tallow Chandlers Hall in the City of London in honour of Lawrence's 25 years as Chairman of the British Diabetic Association. Some 70 past and present members of the Council attended, along with family friends and overseas colleagues. All the Lawrence family were present, including his brother, Dr George Lawrence. Sir Basil Henriques presided, and others present included Sir Henry Dale, Dr George Graham, Professor F. G. Young, Professor J. P. Hoet, Dr F. Gerritzen and Mr Pieter Duys. The toast to Lawrence was proposed by J. P. McNulty, Honorary Secretary of the BDA:

We have come together to-night to do homage to Doctor Lawrence. All of us in this room, or practically all, have been helped by him and many hundreds of thousands outside of this gathering have benefited from his medical wisdom and skilled guidance. In fact, the whole diabetic community owes a great deal to our guest, because his work has not been confined to the personal care of his patients, but has spread to diabetics in many lands through his books, his articles, his speeches and through the influence he had had in the field of his specialist choice upon a younger generation of doctors.

To a layman there is generally an aura of mystery that doth hedge the physician. The workings of his own body are but little understood by the ordinary man, nor do they as a rule excite his interest, except of course when he is ill or in pain. Then he tends to seek comfort, alleviation of his forebodings and reassurance. Preferably he seeks them from his doctor. He becomes susceptible to that aura of mystery, which in the main is not a bad thing for there is a therapeutic value to omniscience … and it saves a lot of time in the life of a busy physician.

I do not think however that Lawrence has indulged in high priest craft unduly. When I first consulted him some 25 years or so ago I told him that I had put my business and domestic affairs in order and that I placed myself unreservedly in his hands – a phrase more suitable for addressing the leader of some semi-forlorn hope than a Harley Street consultant. But Lawrence had no use for pseudo-heroics and told me to 'come off it' or words to that effect.

In the years since then I have had many talks with Lawrence and my admiration for his qualities as a doctor, an organiser and as a human being has steadily grown. His international reputation has never gone to his head; his work for diabetic welfare has shown him possessed of deep sympathy, unerring

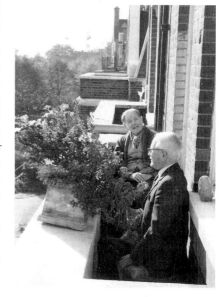

1967 Lawrence and his brother George on the balcony at Sheffield Terrace. This was to be their last meeting.

tact and uncanny skill. Perhaps the finest contribution he has made to the well-being of diabetics was his part, and his was the greatest part, in the formation and development of the organisation which is now known as the British Diabetic Association. Twenty-five years later it all seems so logical, but at the outset it was a novel venture based on the idea that people suffering from the same malady, would, given the opportunity, band together for mutual aid and comfort. Many good

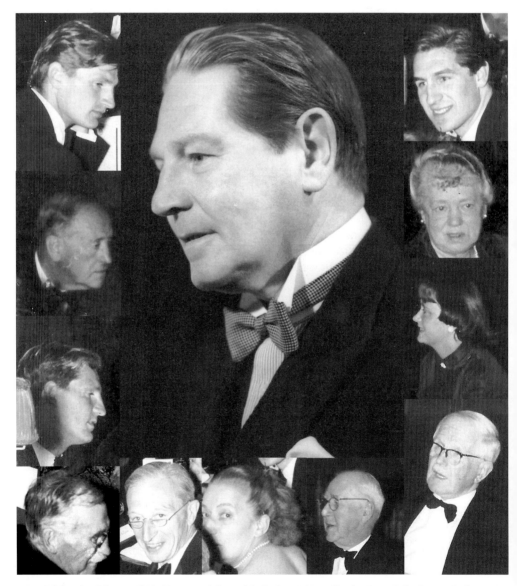

BDA Celebration Dinner, 1959. From top left, anticlockwise: Adam, Charles Best, Rob, George Graham, Lord Harmsworth, Lilian Pearce, Henry Dale, George Lawrence, Clover, Deenah Lawrence, Dan.

ideas die a-borning, but the idea of forming an association of diabetics and those concerned with diabetics did not. It was kept alive at first chiefly by Lawrence's skilful midwifery and was later brought to healthy adulthood by his careful guardianship. Later the idea spread and diabetic associations in many lands followed our lead. The International Diabetes Federation came into being. Naturally, Lawrence became its first president.

If ever a monument is needed for Lawrence, we can say paraphrasing the dedication in St. Paul's Cathedral to Sir Christopher Wren, 'Look around you.' Over a quarter of a million diabetics in this country and many hundreds of thousands in other lands can pay tribute to this good doctor and this good man. So now, on their behalf, let us drink to Doctor Lawrence and wish him and his devoted wife and family many years of good health and happiness.

A month later, a further dinner was held in the House of Commons, sponsored by Mr (later Sir John) Tilney (1907–94), MP, to celebrate the Association's 25th anniversary. The toast to the Association was proposed by Tilney, and, in reply, Lawrence commented that:

all through dinner he had been thinking of the many speakers who had made after-dinner speeches in that room, and when Mr. Tilney had been speaking, he could not help thinking 'Thank God Tilney is a diabetic.'

Lawrence continued his active interest in all matters concerning the care of diabetics. In June 1961, he wrote to Jim Jackson at the BDA about a visit he had had from a representative of the sole distributor of a new powdered sugar product:

Despite the fact that a Berlin analyst found 85% of invert sugar, these products are highly recommended even to severe diabetics. A pamphlet (written in English) advertising these products contains gross mis-statements. I have myself tested this sugar and confirmed the presence of a large amount of glucose. Other products tested here have given a positive iodine test for starch. The representative alleged that by merely submitting analyses to the Board of Trade permission has been granted for the importation of unlimited supplies from Germany. I gather the products are on sale in 60 'Health Stores' in this country and that it is hoped to interest leading stores. The free use of these products by misguided diabetics could lead to disastrous results and this is an urgent matter for the British Diabetic Association to take up. I know nothing about possible legal implications and you should certainly get legal advice.

Lawrence continued to attend meetings of the Executive Council of the BDA, and of other committees in whose work he was particularly interested, but in 1961 he retired from the Chairmanship after 27 years. Jim Jackson, who had the unenviable duty of asking if he was prepared to continue in office, recalls putting the question to him, and receiving the answer: 'Who could possibly succeed me?' To names of other long-serving medical members of the Council, the comment was 'No!', until the name of Dr B. A. Young, a physician in Greenwich and member of the Socialist Medical Association, was raised:

Ah; he hasn't got a private practice, has he?! An excellent choice.

Young proved in every way a most excellent successor, despite the fact that Lawrence continued to serve as Vice-Chairman, which might have been an embarrassment were it not for Young's considerable tact and good sense. Lawrence was himself appointed as Honorary Life President of the BDA.

He attended meetings of the Medical and Scientific Section, and still attended meetings of BDA Committees, although this virtually ceased when the Association moved from Harley Street to Alfred Place, off Tottenham Court Road. Encouraged by his sons and by Lilian Pearce, he started writing his autobiography, much of which is quoted in the early parts of this volume. His handwriting gradually became slow and laboured, which impeded the flow of his thoughts, and he was often distracted: there are several scrawled starts to articles and stories showing his imaginative and restless mind. He loved writing, and his increasing infirmities, which stemmed the tide of expression, frustrated him deeply.

Lawrence's youngest son Dan and I had both been to Frensham Heights School. We started going out together in the summer of 1963 and Dan introduced me to his parents a few weeks into our relationship. The family lived in a large mansion flat, with a long central corridor. The front rooms overlooked a beautiful communal garden with mature trees. I was led into Lawrence's warm study, which smelt of sherry and of dust on an overheated metal lampshade.

My future father-in-law was sitting on a polished leather swivel chair in front of a large desk. He was wearing a loose, soft old velvet smoking jacket over a wing collar and bow tie. He peered at me with disarming intensity over his half-moon steel-framed spectacles. On his feet he wore scuffed, but oddly dainty, house slippers. His good hand was crossed to hold and repeatedly stroke his palsied one and there was a very strong sense of his presence. He reminded me of Mr Badger from *The Wind in the Willows*.

His desk was set into large black shelving stretched right across one end of the room and was covered with old books and dozens of framed family photographs and also a photograph of his ill-fated friends from the Gordon Highlanders. A

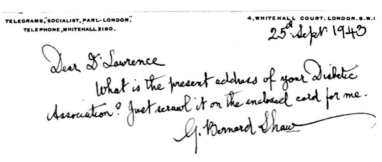

Letter from G. B. Shaw.

battered Anglepoise lamp made a pool of light on his desk, catching the colours in a decanter of red wine and illuminating dancing dust motes. There was a portrait of Beethoven looking striking, intense and not unlike Lawrence himself. A polished bronze head of Voltaire smiled benignly down from a shelf. Papers and notebooks were scattered across the desk.

He spoke with some difficulty, needing to tip his head back and almost roar out the words. At first I was rendered speechless, which was odd for one so garrulous. As an immature 19-year-old who had yet to be liberated by the 1960s, I had no idea how to address him. 'Robin' seemed far too presumptuous. We always addressed male friends of my parents with the 'Uncle' handle, and even at our relatively progressive school, male teachers were called 'Sir'. Neither title seemed the least appropriate for him, yet 'Dr Lawrence' was too formal. In the five years of knowing and then sharing a house with him, I never quite got over this initial stumbling block and always addressed him with a small cough and an awkward 'um er …'.

He was alarmingly direct and brusque in his manner, but this could be offset by a charming twinkle. One needed to choose words carefully, which, being young, gauche and nervous, I found hard to do. Words, so difficult to find at first, just came tumbling out and could be met with a somewhat puzzled, severe and penetrating gaze. At that time, I had no real wisdom or insight into his position or an appreciation of how difficult life had become for him. The stroke had debilitated him severely. Everyone who spoke to me about him started with, 'You should have known him before his stroke … so witty … so lively.' Anna, his devoted wife of 36 years, was unwell with backache. She could only bear minimal physical contact with him. This caused him much distress as he tried to massage her neck and shoulders for her fibrositis.

In that summer of 1963, I would often visit the Lawrence household. I first met Anna at Lords, where we were watching Dan play real tennis. I immediately warmed to her. My fear was that she would be some unapproachable society *grande dame*, but in fact was wonderfully easy, charming and droll. One of our early conversations was about marzipan, which neither of us liked. She told herself that she liked almonds, she liked sugar and that next time she ate marzipan she would simply refer to it as *milled nuts*. I've tried that ever since and it certainly helps. She was constantly mislaying her glasses and would peer around looking for them, muttering that she simply had to take herself in hand. We discovered a mutual interest in Thurber cartoons.

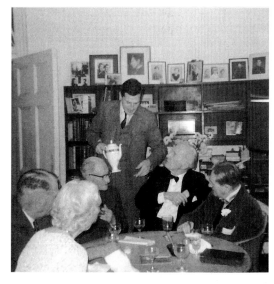

Lawrence in his study, 1965. Adam is serving coffee. Robert Forgan, with spectacles, is by the coffee pot.

In the early years of their marriage, the Lawrences had held rather formal musical soirees after dinner. Before the War, they would even set out gilded chairs for their audience. Such musical gatherings were now held in the large music room in the flat, overlooking the communal gardens, and had become very relaxed and informal. An enormous rubber plant had been trained across the ceiling of the room, and a large replica bust of Hermes of Praxiteles sat on a side table. Anna, who was finding it increasingly difficult to sit upright for any length of time, accompanied me on the piano for a short viola piece. This was the first time I'd ever been accompanied by such a professional; Anna had been Madame Rambert's repetiteur, and I was enchanted by the way she drew out subtleties in the phrasing that had previously passed me by. I'd been accompanied by pianists who made it feel like some sort of competition to see who could shine the brightest and get to the end first, but there was none of this with Anna. Dan would dust off his trumpet, an instrument that he had learned as a boy but had since neglected, and play 'Land of Hope and Glory' vigorously. A retired brigadier from the flat below would sing 'Who is Sylvia' in a pleasant tenor voice. Lawrence was desperate to participate with pieces from his old family *Scottish Students' Song Book* and would restlessly tap his fingers as if playing the piano. It must have been very painful for him to be sidelined when music had played such a central part in his life with Anna.

The love that Lawrence had inspired in his sons was remarkable. Rob, the eldest, was a GP in Kent with a young family, but visited every week. Adam, also a doctor, was working in Paris and could only return home infrequently. Dan, as the only son still at home, had a particular affinity with his father and it was touching to watch them together. Dan had a gift for reading the needs of any invalid. He would support his father in a tender way, gently encouraging him and helping him to wash, sorting out his urine test and putting him to bed, taking infinite care to make him comfortable. Anna was too poorly to do any of this, so a residential nurse was employed, but Dan would often do both the lengthy getting-up procedure at weekends as well as putting him to bed. When the nurse was off duty, Dan would take the greatest care to make his father look immaculate and give him that 'spick and span' feeling that he so appreciated: tie straight, hair first

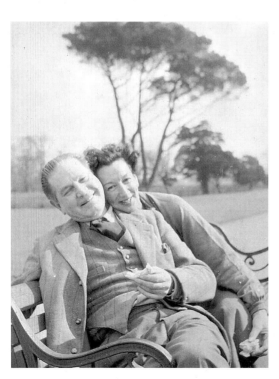
Anna Lawrence, late 1950s.

massaged then beautifully combed back, fresh carnation correctly placed. When we went away at weekends to Hayling, Dan would regularly do physiotherapy on his father's stiff left arm. If Lawrence's bell went off in the night, he was there in an instant to see what was needed. When Dan returned from work, he went straight into the study to chat and laugh with his father over a bottle of South African sherry.

In November of 1963, an old medical friend, Dr Livingstone, visited the family at home and was shocked by Anna's appearance. Lawrence had needed a great deal of care during that autumn. He had had another minor stroke, his diabetes could fly out of control and no one had really noticed just how ill Anna had become. She had had a partial mastectomy 20 years earlier and now had disseminated breast cancer affecting her liver. Anna returned home to be nursed for the remaining few weeks of her life. I was visiting frequently at the time, and Lawrence would burst out tearfully to me that he supposed I had noticed a further deterioration in Anna. Using his stick, he would stumble along into her room, but would find the sight of her dwindling form too distressing, so Dan would lead him away.

Anna died aged 61 in January 1964. Lawrence was utterly distraught and kept saying that he was the one who should have gone. Dan took time off work and they went away to stay with Dino Spranger, Lawrence's old friend from Florence days. Later, when we were married in February 1965, I moved into the flat to live with Dan, Lawrence and a procession of resident nurses, some of whom have remained lifelong friends and others who were quite a trial to live with at the time. The early months of the marriage provided a rigorous training for me in domestic science. Dan came back early from work for the first week after our return from honeymoon to teach me how to cook. He found a most willing pupil, since I quickly discovered that I loved cooking – which was handy as Lawrence liked to have a simple three course meal on the table at exactly 7.30 pm as he always injected his insulin at 7.20 pm.

Lawrence's sister-in-law, Gwen Batson, came up once a week to spend the day with him, and his cousin from Aberdeen, Sheila Kerr-Smith, came over from King's, where she was a ward sister, to have supper with him and talk about Aberdeen and the family. His dear friend Esther Boumphrey was another faithful visitor. He loved her wit and imagination. She was the author of *Hoojibahs and Humans*, a charming and whimsical story for children. She also had a talent for making beautiful table decorations: her clever, mosaic fairy has been gracing the Lawrence Christmas tree for over 60 years. Lawrence also enjoyed nothing better than an informal supper in his study with old friends and colleagues. A large dinner with his old friends was held in November 1967 to celebrate his 75th birthday.

Lawrence continued to see patients at his Harley Street practice until 1966, but by that time it was really the ever-loyal Lilian Pearce who ran the practice. Although colleagues privately thought that he should have bowed out much earlier, and some rather unkindly referred to the partnership as Dr Pearce and Mr Lawrence, it meant a very great deal to him to dress up smartly ready to be driven up to Harley Street twice a week by the excellent caretaker Arthur Watkins and see his patients. Although he came back exhausted, he found it stimulating and enjoyable, and testaments from his patients showed how they appreciated his continuing care. A note from Dan to Lilian Pearce in May 1966 told her:

We had an excellent weekend at Hayling and Dad did a lot of walking. He is pretty mobile and in good spirits but seems a little off balance sometimes when he first stands up. He is looking forward to coming in on Wednesday and Thursday. I gather he was in a very obstructive mood last Thursday, which means he was probably recognising that something was wrong but was getting better. I do hope he isn't being too difficult.

Lawrence's last publication was a letter in the *Lancet* on 17 June 1967,[6] based entirely on his own experience and seeking, as always, an answer to a problem. He was curious to explore a possible connection between hypoglycaemia and the onset of neurological problems in a hemiplegic limb. Composing the letter caused him much difficulty, since by this time his movements had become uncoordinated and his handwriting was very wavering.

In the summer of 1967, Lawrence was the subject of a leading article in *The*

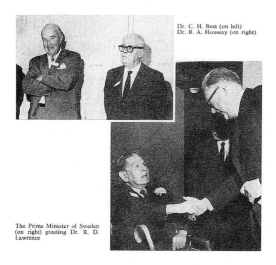

Dr. C. H. Best (on left)
Dr. B. A. Houssay (on right)

The Prime Minister of Sweden (on right) greeting Dr. R. D. Lawrence

In 1967, Lawrence, accompanied by his son Dan, travelled to Sweden to attend what would be his last IDF Congress.

Times Diary commenting on his forthcoming visit to Stockholm for the Sixth IDF Congress. There, in a wheelchair, escorted by Dan, and wearing the signature carnation in his buttonhole, he was warmly greeted by many old friends. Margaret Best recorded in her diary:

6th IDF conference – attended by 2000 delegates. Charles Best, Joseph Hoet, Bernardo Houssay and Robin Lawrence all past presidents of the IDF were on the platform.

A group of them went to hear some opera:

Dan Lawrence and I teased him afterwards by saying that he should have sung a note or two while he was up there.

With Lilian Pearce's help, Lawrence wrote to Charles Best on 23 October 1967:

Although we met in Stockholm and I was glad to see you so well, we had not much time to talk together. I particularly want to know what the men in Toronto and Canada in general think of Loubatières* claim in the Banting Memorial lecture (given at KCH on Friday October 6th) that the sulphonamides increase the size of the islets of Langerhans and hence insulin production. Has anybody but Loubatières proved this to the satisfaction of the medical profession as a whole? It certainly hasn't impressed me in that way.

There's no urgency about this question, but I would like to know please.

Unlike some of his colleagues and contemporaries, Lawrence was never honoured. Lack of it never bothered him. An honorary degree was bestowed on him by the University of Toronto, but he was never knighted. It appears from family memory that he was twice offered a knighthood but refused. Dan recalls at least two occasions hearing his mother tut affectionately when a telephone request for a ticket or some booking was refused by saying, 'If you'd accepted that knighthood, we'd have got the table!' Another suggestion is that once, when a royal visitor was touring the wards at King's, Lawrence kept her waiting as he was dealing with an emergency case and that, if royal feathers are ruffled, the chances of receiving a knighthood are then minimized.

Lawrence clung tenaciously to his increasingly difficult life, with all the limitations and indignities imposed by the stroke. He had always been one to say that, as a medical man with the means at his disposal, he would finish himself off swiftly if disability ever struck – but this was not possible. Although his cognitive function remained unimpaired, he was lonely and could never get comfortable at night. Those last years were busy ones for us, with a young family, but now,

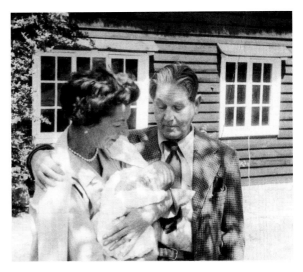

Lawrence and Anna with their first grandchild, Jonathan, born 1960.

---

* August Loubatières (1912–1977) was a French physiologist who discovered the insulin secreting action of a new sulphonamide during The Second World War.

having spent so much time researching the early part of his life and having come to understand his achievements, I would give anything to sit in the study that I rather avoided then, and have a conversation about his family, the Aberdeen days, India, Kashmir and the Gulmarg, and about his friends, and discuss every aspect of his life and have him tell me more about LandsB, Jack Mason, Robert Forgan, H. G. Wells, George Bernard Shaw, and the army of friends, patients and colleagues who had marched through his life.

He was a fond grandfather to Rob and Clover's children and also to Anna-Louise and then to Hugo, but increasingly he found it harder to be with small children. He became very frail and unstable, needing inpatient treatment at King's on several occasions.

One afternoon in late August 1968, when his nurse had gone out, I settled Lawrence down for his afternoon rest, covered him with a rug and left him to sleep. Later, he called for some water and was a little testy with me, but somehow I did not say what was uppermost in my mind. I wanted to berate him and plead with him to be more reasonable with the troupe of resident nurses who kept handing in their resignation, but a divine hand of restraint intervened. Instead, I suggested he look up at the treetops in the garden and watch the sun play on the leaves. He later slipped into unconsciousness and died in his sleep. After 45 years of insulin, the 'splendid life', as he liked to call it, ended.

Later, his three sons gathered. They dressed him in his pinstriped suit, placed a fresh carnation in his buttonhole and brushed his hair. All his favourite photographs were set about around him, including a treasured one of Anna, and together the brothers cracked a bottle of whisky and sat talking and reminiscing beside their father for the whole evening. It was more of a quartet than a trio, and it seemed entirely natural. It was my first experience of a death, and to this day not a detail of it has vanished from my mind. It seemed such a proper and sensible way for sons to be with their father, talking, laughing and shedding tears on his last night in his home.

The memorial service held in the chapel at KCH two months after his death and was a splendid gathering of friends, family and colleagues. Professor Frank Young gave an address which encompassed Lawrence's life, achievements, personality and qualities.

Some of Lawrence's ashes were scattered at the base of a silver birch tree in the garden at Saltings to join those of his beloved Anna. The tree had been planted by their sons in 1953 to celebrate their parents' silver wedding anniversary. A few years after Lawrence's death, Dan and I took the children for a holiday near Aberdeen. We shared a small cottage with Lawrence's nephew Tam and family and we saw many of the places Lawrence had known as a child. We visited those cousins May and Sheila Kerr-Smith mentioned fondly in his letters from India during The First World War. They were by now venerable elderly women and no longer those children whom he urged should be taken down to the beach and given the freedom to play.

On a bright sunny day we took his ashes to a Deeside bridge and after a slightly unfortunate misunderstanding about which way the wind was actually blowing, we scattered them in the broad and fast flowing river where he'd landed so many fine fish. We watched the current take them down towards Aberdeen and slowly out to the grey North Sea.

References

1. As set out by the Charity Commission scheme of 1892 for the triennial award. It appears that for some time the Council has not set an essay question.
2. From an article based on a paper read at a meeting of the Medical Society of London, on the occasion of the award of the Fothergillian Medal to Sir Francis Avery Jones in 1980.
3. Lawrence RD. Reading and writing about new diseases. *Br Med J* 1955; **i**: 286.
4. Phenylketonuria (PKU) is a rare condition in which a baby is born without the ability to properly break down an amino acid called phenylalanine.
5. Byssinosis is a disease of the lungs brought on by breathing in cotton dust or dusts from other vegetable fibres such as flax, hemp or sisal while at work.
6. Lawrence RD. Hemiplegia in a diabetic producing unilateral peripheral neuritis and hypoglycemic attacks. *Lancet* 1967; **289**: 1321–2.

Index

Page numbers in *italics* indicate a photograph. RDL = Lawrence, Robert Daniel (Robin)

Greeves, Reginald Affleck 125
guanidine compounds 194
Guest, Major Oscar 95

H
haemochromatosis 128–9
Hagedorn, Hans Christian 121–2
Haire, Dr Norman 108
Haldane Report 95
Hardwick, Christopher 179
Harley, George 1
Harmsworth, Lord *212*
Harris, Harry 97
Harrison, Geoffrey Arthur 4
    publications 84, 85, 192
    supporting RDL 96
    telegraph to RDL regarding insulin 12–13, *13*
    wanting insulin trials 7
Haydon, Dr Leonard 111, 116, 117–19
Hayling Island home 111–13
Hoet, Professor J. P. 165, *209, 209*
Hogben, Lancelot 97
Hunt, John A. 187
Hutton Residential School 144
hyperglycaemia 122
hypoglycaemia 90-2, 124, 197, 218

I
IDF *see* International Diabetes Foundation
India, RDL in 63–78
Inge, William Ralph 10
Inkster, Walter 32, 44, 51
insulin
    actions of 192–3
    availability in Britain 12
    costs 87, 90
    discovery 2, 6
    dosage 84
        balancing 87–8, 191–2
        exercise and 91
        for ketoacidosis 196–7
    early trials 6–10, 10, 81–2
    endocrine effects on 193
    false remedies and abuses of 194–5
    GP supervision 91–2
    injections 82–3, 121–2, 183
    other uses 96
    panic buying in WWII 129–30
    potency 84
    preparations 84
    protamine 122
    protamine zinc (PZI) 122–3
    resistance 193
    sensitivity 127
    syringe *15*, 84

    types 121–2
    see also blood sugar
Insulin Leo Retard 121–2
insulin phototungstate 194–5
insuline 2
International Diabetes Foundation (IDF)
    Congresses 166–7
    congresses 174–7, 209, 218–19
    Executive Board 173
    foundation 165–6, 170
    Member Associations 175
    RDL as President 165–6
    South African application to join 176–7
islet cells regeneration 84

J
Jackson, J. G. L. (Jim) 146, 147, 179, 213
Jeanneret, F. C. A. *209*
Jeffery, Ed 6–7
Jock's Society 51
Jordan, Helen 186–7
Joslin, Elliott Proctor 3, 82, 85, 117, 166–7, 196

K
Kerr-Smith, Sheila 217
ketoacidosis 196–7
Keun, Odette 109, *110*
Kinfaun's Castle, RMS (Castle Line) 61–3, *62*
King's College Hospital *81*
    bed shortages 4, *4*
    diabetic clinic 94–5, 136
    RDL colleagues *184*
    see also under Lawrence, Robert: appointments

L
lag storage curve 200
Laing, Hugh *105*, 112–13
Lancereaux, Etienne 1
Landsborough Thomson, (Sir) Arthur 7, 41–2, 55, 56, 57–8
Lawrence
    Adam Gay (RDL's son) 173, *212, 215*
        birth 110
        childhood memories 112–13
        hobbies 114
        as teenager 155
    Ann (RDL's grandmother) *19*
    Anna (RDL's wife) *107, 172*
        death 217
        early life 102, *114*
        family history 101–2
        holidays in Cornwall 154
        illness 215, 217
        involvement with Beltane School 152–3
        love of music 107, 153, 216